OUR HUMAN HEARTS

Literature and Medicine
MARTIN KOHN AND CAROL DONLEY, EDITORS

Our
Human Hearts

❧

A Medical and Cultural Journey

❧

By Albert Howard Carter III

❧

The Kent State

University Press

KENT, OHIO

❧

© 2006 by The Kent State University Press, Kent, Ohio 44242

ALL RIGHTS RESERVED

Library of Congress Catalog Card Number 2005021205

ISBN-13: 978-0-87338-863-4

Manufactured in the United States of America

10 09 08 07   5 4 3 2

Library of Congress Cataloging-in-Publication Data

Carter, Albert Howard, 1943–

Our human hearts : a medical and cultural journey / by Albert Howard Carter III.

p.   cm. — (Literature and medicine series ; 3)

ISBN-13: 978-0-87338-863-4 (pbk. : alk. paper) ∞

ISBN-10: 0-87338-863-1 (pbk. : alk. paper) ∞

1. Heart—Diseases—Popular works.   2. Heart—Mythology.   3. Heart in literature.

I. Title.   II. Literature and medicine (Kent, Ohio) ; 3.

RC682C48 2006   616.1'2—dc22   2005021205

British Library Cataloging-in-Publication data are available.

Contents

ɠ෨

Acknowledgments

⸙

I WISH to thank many people who made, directly and indirectly, this book possible.

First, I thank my hosts at the Institute of Medicine and Humanities, a cooperative venture of St. Patrick Hospital and the University of Montana, in Missoula, Montana, particularly Jan Willms, the former director, and Dixie McLaughlin, the coordinator/administrator during my stay. I also thank Lawrence L. White Jr., the then CEO of St. Patrick Hospital, and George M. Dennison, president of the University of Montana, Missoula. I also thank Bruce Bigley and Lois M. Welch, successive chairs of the Department of English at U of M, where I taught a course on literature and medicine. I thank members of the board and advisory board for the institute for making my semester in Missoula possible.

I thank Gerry Brenner, professor in the English department, for many kindnesses, and also his wife Terry. Thanks to Albert Borgmann, who invited me to address the Philosophy Club on the topic of hearts and who provided me with the Thomas Jefferson passage. I thank Dixie and Gary McLaughlin for their support and friendship; I thank Jane Rectanwald and Fran Weigand for their friendship and many a good hike around the Missoula area. I thank Steve Oreskovich, the rector of Holy Spirit Parish, and the parishioners for many kindnesses; my wife and I sang in the chancel choir directed by Nancy Cooper and attended a supper club that provided fellowship and hilarity.

I thank all members of my class "The Physician in Literature" at the U of M. I enjoyed their interest in health and disease, healing and dying, and their good humor and patience in educating me, a flatlander, in Rocky Mountain lore.

The International Heart Institute of Montana, Missoula, was crucial to my research. I thank Drs. Carlos M. G. Duran and James H. Oury, scientists David Cheung and David Pang, research nurse Katie Mackey, and administrator Carole V. Erickson.

I thank many others who aided my research: Michael Kevin Curry, Jayne and Kevin Curry, Paulette Parpart, Steve Oreskovich, George Meese, and Johnnie and Zelma Reddick. Also physicians Joseph Knapp and Gary Grant. I thank Manfred Thurmann, M.D., of the Academy of Senior Professionals at Eckerd College and James R. Foster, M.D., a clinical professor of medicine and cardiology, University of North Carolina School of Medicine and a practicing cardiologist in Raleigh, N.C., for review of some of the more technical chapters; any errors remaining are my own. I thank various technicians, nurses, and many patients, including members of a Mended Hearts Club, for informal conversation that enrich the book. I thank Doug Harrell, Pastoral Care, Bayfront Medical Center, and Sandy Giles, parish nurse.

I thank Richard Croudt, Carrboro, N.C., for preparing the illustrations for this book.

I thank physicians Allan Gabster, Richard Oldenski, Andrew J. Peterson, Eugene P. Orringer, Carolyn Sidor, Arthur Axelbank, Jane Arbuckle Petro, and Carolyn Becker for information and/or support. I thank the medical librarians at Bayfront Medical Center, St. Patrick Hospital, the University of South Florida, the University of North Carolina, Chapel Hill, and Duke University. I thank the St. Petersburg branch of the American Heart Association for many materials; these are free and available to anyone.

From my previous home institution, Eckerd College, I thank Dean of Faculty Lloyd Chapin for making my Montana sojourn possible. Eckerd professors who helped me with linguistic or scientific detail include Professors Julienne H. Empric, Gary E. Melzer, Cynthia Totten, Nanette Nascone-Yoder, Bill and Vivian Parsons, Guy Bradley, Olivia McIntyre, and David J. Bryant. I thank my faithful and lively work scholars, Heather Furrow and Megan Rita Kelleher. I thank all my colleagues—faculty and students alike—for friendship and intellectual stimulation.

I thank the following for discussion about this topic and, in many cases, reading portions of the manuscript: Mary Ann Willis, Rebecca Alice Carter, Nancy Corson Carter, and Colleen Adomaitis. I also thank Carolyn and Lloyd Horton, Susan and T. J. Gill, Tom and Marian Price, George and Karen Meese, Bruce and Carol Hewitt, Trish and Bob Berrett, Jimmy and Delores Carter, Barbara Barr and Jerry Gershenhorn, Al and Janet Rabil, Carl and Janet Edwards, Ruth Hamilton, Doris and Jim Tippens, Norm and Nancy Gustaveson, Mark and Allison Davidson, and Betty and Jerry Eidenier for their friendship and support.

For a visiting appointment that allowed me to give undivided attention to the finishing of the book, I thank Dr. Desmond K. Runyan, chair, Department of Social Medicine, University of North Carolina, Chapel Hill, and other members and staff of the department for their colleagueship.

I thank my editors of the Literature and Medicine Series, Carol Donley and Martin Kohn (both of Hiram College).

I thank members of my immediate family: Nancy Corson Carter, wife; Rebecca Alice Carter, daughter; Avise Nissen, sister; and Marjorie Dargan Carter, mother. Their love and support can never be adequately acknowledged.

Haunted by Hearts

When I was at Emory University, I observed first-year medical students dissecting their cadavers; one of the most dramatic events was the removal of a heart from a large opening in the chest, a scene described in *First Cut: A Season in the Anatomy Lab* (New York: Picador, 1997). The first student to have a heart free from a body invited me to touch it and hold it in the palm of my hand. As I hefted this strange object—heavy in its meat, light in its four chambers—I wondered how it worked and why humans had made it for thousands of years a symbol of love, courage, spirit, and, of course, mortality. Another student showed me the heart of a man who had died from a heart attack. "See, the tissue below [the point of blockage] all died without oxygen," she said. "Killed him."

Such impressions visual, tactile, olfactory—have stayed with me, even haunted me, for years. What is this wondrous organ that beats in our chests? How does it contribute to our physical lives, our imaginative lives, our intuitive lives? A professor of literature, I began to collect heart phrases ("heartfelt," "brokenhearted," "heart of gold") and literary uses of the heart. Even as far back as *The Epic of Gilgamesh*, roughly five thousand years ago, humans were interested in hearts. We have described the heart in many ways, from the emotional to the cellular, from the medical to the spiritual.

Two other events spurred me on. One was a series of minor chest pains, mild enough that I didn't seek medical help—although perhaps I should have. But I told myself the pains were a manifestation of some general anxiety or stress at work. Or maybe as I read about heart health and heart illness—my version of the med student's "sophomore syndrome"—I imagined that I suffered from each disease I read about. Whatever the causes, the discomfort in my chest emphasized in a personal and visceral way the central importance of the heart. I thought of my grandmother, who had been a heart patient. As a youth I knew her as loving and kind, but also weak, timorous, and moody. Was this to be my future? Treatments are better now than in her day, but still about one half of Americans die of cardiovascular disease: it's our Number One Killer. In the course of writing this book, in fact, severe chest pains sent me to the hospital.

The second (and more happy) event was my appointment to a distinguished professorship in medical humanities in a joint program between St. Patrick Hospital and the University of Montana, Missoula. My responsibilities were to teach one class at the university (in literature and medicine), to offer a series of town-gown seminars at the hospital (on hearts, of course), and to do research. To my good fortune, two floors above my office at the hospital was the International Heart Institute of Montana. This institute was very helpful in providing me with much background and the particular foreground of a patient, Michael, whose story opens this narrative. As the beautiful Montana autumn wore on, it became clear to me that the heart was at the center of a classic problem: is the heart merely an organ (a problem in ontology), or is it an object perceived only through the viewpoint(s) of the observer (a problem in epistemology)? The answer, this book will attempt to show, is an interactive one: yes, the heart exists in humans and other animals as a vital organ, but we know it only through a series of lenses—biological, medical, linguistic, emotional, spiritual, and so forth. Even a lack of awareness of the heart and its health (as in unhealthy lifestyles) is a way of dealing with the heart.

What Is the Heart?

Cardiologist and poet John Stone has suggested that there are two hearts within each of us, the literal organ that pumps blood and a metaphorical one, a symbolic center that houses our emotions, our highest values, even our souls. Stone calls the metaphoric heart "an extra dimension" to the literal heart (see his introduction to *In the Country of Hearts*, New York: Delacorte, 1990). Gail Godwin, in her highly personal *Heart* (New York: William Morrow, 2000) suggests that these two hearts suffered "The Great Heart Split of the Seventeenth Century," when William Harvey explained how the heart is a pump. I'm suggesting in this book that the meanings of the heart, whether medical or cultural, are all metaphoric, and that they are many—sometimes conflicting, sometimes overlapping, and often changing—within each of us, especially if we have chest pains or experience any kind of heart illness. Medical perspectives of the heart are metaphoric, creating models that selectively represent aspects of the heart. I will compare the medical metaphors with the metaphors of the wider culture (valentines, the Sacred Heart of Jesus, various words and phrases) to see how each may illuminate the other and to explore the varying distances between the two poles, which I will call "medical" and "cultural." These terms are inexact, of course, since medicine has its own culture (or subculture) and people in medicine are also within the larger culture.

While there is some truth to C. P. Snow's famous (notorious?) lecture about the two cultures of the sciences and the humanities, persons delivering health care in particular are usually trained to respond to both the biological and the personal needs of patients. Whether they can always deliver both levels of care may depend on other factors, but training in communication, ethics, and patients' anxieties are now routine.

I'll expand Stone's sense of metaphor to include ways biologists and physicians perceive the heart. A metaphor, we recall, is a simile—"He was a man like a mountain"—with the "like" or "as" repressed: "He was a mountain of a man." A metaphor suggests an overlap between two fields, a point of similarity, so that the man in this example is somehow mountain-like. (The Greek root *metapherein* still makes sense, *to transfer.*) We perceive, usually subconsciously, an *image*—the sight of a mountain, or perhaps even the physical labor involved in climbing a mountain, which we carry across to this man. In literary studies, an image is an appeal to sense (sight, touch, etc.), so that a visceral perception is simulated in our imaginations. Perhaps it is only a ripple in our consciousness, but from it we sense connotations of value, such as (in this example) power, durability, and size. Metaphors are selective, bringing some attributes into focus while hiding others. They are a map, not the territory, but we sometimes see them as the territory, especially if we forget the nature of metaphors. "Ah, here's Mrs. Schultz," a radiologist said one day in the reading room as a set of X-ray studies came into his hands. He didn't mean it literally, but for the moment, and for his professional role, the X-ray films before him *were* Mrs. Schultz.

Metaphors pervade medicine. The patient has a metaphoric parallel in the chart; where the in-take complaint, history, lab results, and progress notes are all selective models of what is assumed equal to the patient's state of being. (See my "Esthetics and Anesthetics: Mimesis, Hermeneutics, and Treatment in Literature and Medicine," *Literature and Medicine* 5 [1986]: 141–51.) Samuel Shem's novel *The House of God: A Novel* (New York: R. Marek, 1978) offers this satiric advice: treat the chart, not the patient. And yet doctors know that lab results can be wrong and that X-rays can have "artifacts," representations of light that have no reference to the patient's tissues. Thus in some instances doctors are aware of the limitations of the metaphors before them. In general, though, the modern medical definitions have become specialized and routinized into a world of their own, well beyond the ken of a layperson. On the other hand, physicians can explain heart attacks or congestive heart failure to patients and their families—often in readily perceived metaphors of pumps and plumbing. The medical definitions are ever evolving, of course, as new research provides new models, new treatments, and new influences on cardiac health (epidemiology and alternative medicine, for example). The scientific metaphors have become more and more specific, carrying fewer and fewer wider meanings. Numbers, graphs, and radiological films carry a one-to-one sense of sufficiently accurate—if selective—meanings.

In contrast, the wider cultural values that we see in heart metaphors have become diffuse and idiomatic to the point that we have largely lost the anchoring image of the heart itself, the organ continuously beating in our chests. "Heartfelt," "home is where the heart is," "wear my heart on my sleeve," and scores of other words and phrases flow through our language, scarcely reminding us of our actual hearts. And yet the values suggested in these words and phrases are still important to us. I shall speculate that the loss of our sense of our physical hearts is one source of not only poor health habits but also a lack of meaning in our lives.

Metaphors and their implied values can be brought to explicit consciousness. Critics and commentators often describe, analyze, and critique the metaphors that pervade advertising, politics, and religion as rhetorical strategies aimed to persuade us and move us to action. (Recent examples include President Bush's early use of the term "crusade" and the military's suggestion of the term "Infinite Justice" as the code name for American military action following the September 11 attacks; as their metaphoric meanings were analyzed and made explicit, both were dropped.) When I say I am "haunted" by hearts, I'm suggesting some hidden ghost that invades my consciousness without my permission. I need to examine this metaphor and exorcise it or domesticate it.

What is the heart? The answers will depend on the observer, the generation, and the culture. Humans from ancient times have interpreted the heart in many ways: as the home of the soul, the seat of love, the place of wisdom and justice, the symbol of our vitality. No other human organ has had as many meanings attached to it. We speak of someone as *having the guts to do something,* and we say that someone *is a real brain;* there's also *a man of his kidney* and *to be thin-skinned* and *to have the nerve to do something,* but these are scattered instances compared to over a hundred heart-related phrases in contemporary English. Many survive from earlier languages and cultures: "Create in me a clean heart, O God," the psalmist wrote in ancient times. Why has the heart had such linguistic currency for so many years? Probably because heartbeats symbolize life by their presence, death by their absence. Knowledge of the circulation of blood didn't come until the seventeenth century, but people of earlier times could tell that the presence or absence of breathing and heartbeats was the surest sign of life or death. Further, a rapid heartbeat showed physical effort and emotional turmoil—be it desperate fear or erotic love. If we say, "I'm heartsick," we refer to our emotions, not to the physical organ.

Paradoxically, it is often chest pain or cardiac illness—our own or a family member's or friend's—that renews our interest in the health of the physical heart and perhaps also in our wider sense of the values implied by our uses of the word "heart."

Searching for, Listening to, Hearts

The book's inquiry uses two means of "knowing": searching and listening. *Searching* we're familiar with: it's American, western, scientific. We explore, we follow objectives, we get out there and take action. The geographic setting of my work illustrates this well. On leave from my college in Florida, I traveled to Missoula, Montana, over three thousand miles away. Missoula is a university town of some seventy thousand souls on the west slope of the Rockies, about seventy miles from the Continental Divide. It's a lively place of ranchers, students, aging hippies, artists, and businesspeople; almost everyone enjoys nature throughout four seasons, including the long winter. Lewis and Clark came through this valley on their search for a passage to the Pacific. Even though there are plenty of hearts in Florida, I was too busy to do much with them; ironically, I went a long way to find out about something that resides just below my sternum. In Joseph Campbell's formula of the quest myth, the hero finds a wealth of knowledge and brings it back to his tribe or nation (or readership). Could that be me? I would visit various libraries and labs and talk with various doctors and patients. Medicine seemed to provide the most intense inquiry into the heart; what could I learn from it? But literature and our common speech use symbolic hearts in many ways. I would read extensively and pursue these meanings as well. Such were some of my Active-Scholar inclinations, standard modes of research in this culture.

But as the weeks went by, my wife and I took many a hike in the mountains and valleys around Missoula. It slowly became clear to me that much was to be learned by letting insights occur of their own accord, concepts coming toward the investigator, so to speak, as he or she remains open and attentive. Thus the concept of *listening* became more important to me, as sound waves would come to me. I have a musical background, but also, years ago, I had training as an emergency medical technician; from the latter, I still have a stethoscope, through which I've heard hearts. More speculatively, Peter D. Kramer's book *Listening to Prozac: A Psychiatrist Explores Antidepressant Drugs and the Remaking of the Self* (New York: Penguin, 1994) provided reinforcement here, demonstrating how to take evidence from the culture at large to hear underlying perceptions, values, and expectations. If our hearts are, in some sense, the canaries lowered into the mine shaft of modern life, what can we infer when we notice that about a third of them cause our deaths? There are many factors, of course. Public health and medicine have largely limited death from infectious diseases, so we live longer and experience other ills at a higher rate: cancers, Alzheimer's, Parkinson's, and heart disease. As our population ages, these diseases will increasingly afflict us, our families, and our health-care resources. According to E. Magnus Ohman, a cardiologist leading a nation-wide study of some six hundred hospitals, "During the next decade we are likely to see an overwhelming epidemic of coronary artery disease."

But cardiovascular deaths are already an epidemic. According to the Centers for Disease Control and Prevention, 706,947 deaths in 2002 were attributed to "diseases of heart," our number one killer, with another 161,317 from cerebrovascular illness (largely strokes), our number three killer. Cancer (number two) claimed some 557,256. While the cerebrovascular numbers are about the same for 1995, the heart disease numbers are well down from some 950,000 in 1995, a drop partly attributable to such factors as better diets, increased exercise, and reduced smoking. But still, heart disease is our number one killer. How can we listen to and interpret this epidemic?

Heartbeats themselves well illustrate aspects of perception and interpretation. We typically hear them only if we "go after them" by placing a finger on a pulse, an ear or stethoscope on a chest. (I'm leaving aside a pounding heart that we feel in our own chests after, say, extreme effort.) But what is it that comes toward us as we feel or hear heartbeats? At a physical level, modern biology tells us, heartbeats are waves of energy caused by the opening and closing of the heart valves; these waves spread through the tissues of the chest and outward through the arteries. The pulse we feel in the radial artery at our wrists or in the carotid arteries of our necks are waves "downstream" from the four valves coordinated to keep blood flowing in one direction only. With an ear to the chest, we say we hear a heartbeat, but, more accurately, we sense a sound wave originating in the action of the heart valves, traveling through the chest, and entering our outer ear; this energy is then further converted to mechanical energy in the inner ear, then to the electrical energy that reaches our brain. In short, we don't—we cannot—feel or hear the heart directly, but indirectly—metaphorically, in this discussion—through pulsatile or sound waves which we perceive through our own interpretive physiologies. The pulse at our wrist tells us some two feet downstream how fast the heart is beating. Each wave is, in any absolute sense, old news—but useful news nonetheless; pulse rate and blood pressure are two of the five vital signs routinely taken in every hospital as baseline measures of a person's health. Such metaphoric knowledge permeates cardiology, which uses elaborate methods of interpretation to reach diagnoses and to prescribe treatments. In wider cultural interpretations, heartbeats may signal fear, physical exertion, or romantic excitement. Sometimes we may feel our own hearts beating within our chests after vigorous physical exertion or a strong emotion. This sensation can alarm us or seem normal, depending on how we understand our hearts. We have to know the context in order to interpret the deeper meanings.

Listening is the purposeful reception of noise, bringing to mind a military "listening post" or the "active listening" of counselors. In English, we separate the verb *to listen* from *to hear,* which suggests the reception of sound without purpose. We *hear* noise, but *listen* to a teacher. Cardiologists, ever intentional, listen to not two heartsounds, but four; indeed they can discriminate some two dozen heart problems through careful and intensified listening. (An excellent stethoscope, with three listening elements in a cluster like a flower, can cost three hundred dollars.) The listening, furthermore, has several levels: physical (certain sound waves are perceived), diagnostic (the sounds are interpreted according to medical science), and the more widely symbolic: a thoughtful physician thinks about the total patient, the mortality of all humans, the widest meanings of life. Physician-writer William Carlos Williams felt that much of medicine and literature hinged on listening:

> The poem springs from the half-spoken words of such patients as the physician sees from day to day. He observes it in the peculiar, actual conformations in which its life is hid. Humbly he presents himself before it and by long practice he strives as best he can to interpret the manner of its speech. In that the secret lies. This, in the end, comes perhaps to be the occupation of the physician after a lifetime of careful listening. (*Autobiography* [New York: Random House, 1951], chap. 42).

If we listen to the cultural heart as well as the physical heart, what poem can we imagine about the inner nature of humanity? How can we better overlap the two traditions, medical and literary?

About fifteen years ago I participated in a human growth workshop; the only thing I remember from that day was a conversation I was directed to undertake. Pairs of us were to sit on the floor, place a hand on the other's heart, and share what was important to us. Once linked heart-to-heart, we began our conversations. Although the details of what my partner and I said have left me, the image of closeness, trust, and sharing is still vivid. The exercise was an embodiment of many phrases we use: *to share what's in one's heart, a heart-to-heart talk, taking something to heart.* What if diplomats, labor negotiators, lawyers—any pair of conversationalists—were to talk, hands to hearts?

This book is an attempt to put into dialogue the two major domains of heart interpretation, the biomedical world of modern science, and the cultural (including linguistic and literary) heritage that shapes, even without our conscious awareness, the ways we see and live with our hearts. For C. P. Snow, these were two cultures that had, unfortunately, gone down two different paths. The reasons are easy to see. In modern times, the biomedical world has become so highly specialized that laypeople can't read its technical literature, while the wider cultural language of hearts has become a vague baggage of unexamined images that we take for granted, often forgetting the wisdom it can provide.

Four Heart Patients

I draw on the experiences of four heart patients, who graciously shared with me medical and personal details of their health history. (A note on confidentiality: These four patients and their families gave permission for my use of their stories; other patients described in the book have had the details of their stories changed or are composites so that none can be recognized.) For each, medical science develops an assessment of their cardiac experience, and they develop new understandings of their hearts based on what they learn from doctors, but also based on what they prize most in the wider culture. Michael, a twenty-seven-year-old athlete, is concerned with the basic structures and functions of the heart. Highly verbal, he brings language to bear on his leaking heart valve. Michael's medical treatment is surgical, a direct and dramatic intervention that assumes a knowledge of the structure and functioning of the heart; Michael comes to terms with his heart and also with his family and other persons supporting him. His section explores the terms, both medical and cultural, that we use for the heart, and their implications. His section is the longest, a foundation of information and themes that extend into the next three sections.

Kay's illness, by contrast, is chronic, and her treatment is pharmaceutical, not surgical. The failings of her heart at a cellular level limit its function, and cardiology seeks to shore up the biochemistry to make it work as efficiently as possible. To see her through her continuing troubles, Kay creates (and lives out) various stories that give her life order and meaning; for her, the unlikely pair of yoga and rodeo provides the context for this meaning. In particular, rodeo offers primal, exemplary stories that metaphorically parallel her trials.

For Steve, cardiac illness was caused (at least in part) by pervasive stress, and epidemiology is one of the medical approaches that illuminate his dilemma. He finds that his life has been governed by hidden stories, which he must root out and rewrite in order to live a healthy life. Interventional radiology can show the blockages in his coronary arteries and even remove them in a mechanical operation, but Steve's reassessment of his deepest values and related behaviors becomes the "solid ground" he needs to reduce stress in his life.

Our last patient, Johnnie, is ninety-one years old. He has survived various kinds of heart trouble over several decades; nursed by his wife, he now maintains his health through a version of alternative medicine that includes a spiritual dimension. For him, the words, images, and rituals of religious life are the deepest interpreters and sustainers of his life on earth—and even of a life to come.

These four sections are cumulative on two levels. The first level—the internal, largely medical inquiry—starts with the physical heart and moves outward to more abstract models of the heart: the biochemical functions of the heart, the cultural components of behavior that can cause or contribute to an unhealthy heart, and, finally, the spiritual dimensions of living with a heart.

The second level is the more cultural level in which we start with words and phrases, then move on to various stories, both explicit and implicit, and, finally, to images that succinctly and suggestively define the heart. This is the symbolic, social approach from outside the body, so to speak, as we try to come to terms with the heart, culturally and individually.

While creating my own metaphoric models, I also look at images, starting with a four-square diagram of the heart (a "napkin schematic," page 12). As the book proceeds, I develop a less Cartesian and more dialectical model of the heart (an Alcove Model, pp. 118, 153, 191).

As my Montana semester progressed, as we went for hikes, as I talked with physicians and patients, two further themes emerged as larger contexts: nature and spirituality. Nature was no surprise, indeed it was most obvious. Deer walked through our yard; two bears wandered onto campus. The deer, the bears, and all the other wildlife around us had hearts, and the atomic elements of these hearts were the same as the elements in glacial moraines, forests, and even the complex geology of the Rocky Mountains all around us. What advantages might there be in seeing our hearts as part of nature?

Spiritual aspects were a surprise, in part because it has been "politically correct" in many circles not to mention such things. But all four of these heart patients—people who had looked mortality squarely in the eye—and even some of the doctors mentioned spiritual concerns. Furthermore, spiritual traditions of many sorts use the heart as a symbol.

The specific aims of this book are (1) to explore the various meanings of the heart—biological, medical, psychological, cultural, and spiritual—and to show how these meanings may conflict or overlap; (2) to analyze and critique the separations of the heart's various "meanings," specifically how our denial of the heart has contributed to its neglect through our lifestyles, attitudes, and emotions; and (3) to consider ways we can heal our hearts by reassembling some of the deepest meanings of hearts.

Some years ago I asked Rick, my doctor, whether I was at risk for cancer. Looking over my chart, which included my family medical history, he said, "You're not any more at risk than anyone else." Then he added with a smile, "Statistically speaking, heart will probably get you. It's our number one, grand champion killer." I should add that he and I have a jocular relationship, but his comment broke a taboo and shocked me. Yes, the papers talk about heart disease, but we assume it's always Other People who will so die. But the fact is, whether the heart is the primary cause of death (as in a heart attack) or whether it stops secondary to another cause (such as cancer, emphysema, or severe trauma), we are all mortal, and our hearts will fail all of us sooner or later. (When nosy people asked my physician grandfather, Albert, the cause of one of his patient's death, he'd simply say, "The heart stopped beating.") Although some observers think the number of deaths attributed to heart failure is inflated—it can be an all-too-easy, or "wastebasket" diagnosis—it's undeniable that there will be *a last heartbeat for each of us.* Our culture largely ignores the notion that having a heart means being mortal. In Leo Tolstoy's powerful novella *The Death of Ivan Ilyich* (1896), Ivan suffers greatly from "the lie" that he is not mortally ill, that people do not die.

I have found the human heart to be utterly fascinating. Am I still haunted by it? Perhaps so, but the threatening ghosts have been replaced with more kindly spirits. In this book I shall argue that to accept and celebrate our hearts—with their ultimate, mortal limitations, but also with all their wonderful strengths and symbolic resonances—is the healthiest way to perceive and enjoy them.

The Workings of Michael's Heart

CARDIAC STRUCTURE, CARDIAC FUNCTION

THE MOST HEARTS I've ever seen at once were in a large container in Houston, at the Baylor College of Medicine. We visiting professors were touring an anatomy lab, gaping at all the strange sights. In a big pot maybe eighteen inches high, with straight sides of clear glass, were six, eight, a dozen—who could tell?—hearts stacked on top of each other, like huge olives in a jar. But these hearts were clearly dark, meaty, even brooding, or so it seemed—somewhat purplish-red, with bands of yellow-gray fat on the surface. What sense could we make of them? What did they mean? What stories could they tell? Each heart represented a dead person, as well as the live person who had performed some dramatic act of evisceration. Although we were supposed to be reviewing the anatomy of the lower extremity, the leg, we were entranced by this big pot of hearts. Our guide—an anatomy professor—noticed our distraction and fished out a heart with his bare hand. He showed us the basic features. Since someone had cut slits into the heart muscle, he could give us glimpses of the chambers and valves inside. We stood in silent awe of the ingenious design, knowing that a similar organ was at work, day and night, in our own chests. Just how long could this complex structure work? Might my heart end up like this one?

Later, as we looked at the muscles and tendons of the leg, our guide said something like, "And one day I was speaking to the med students about the medial attachments of the leg and I said—in all my *ex cathedra* glory—that men could sometimes do the splits . . . you know, sitting on the floor with one leg straight forward and the other leg back . . . but only women could do the *side* splits, with each leg out to the side, because of the way their pelvises were constructed. As I paused for a moment one of the male students around these tables said, 'Excuse me, I don't think that's quite accurate.' 'What do you mean?' I said. 'Well, if I can take a minute,' he said, and he stretched one way and another. Then we all watched as he slowly sank to the floor, with one foot going out to the side, and the other going out to the other side in a perfect side split. It turned out he had been a gymnast in college and had developed this

11

flexibility. I thought about this a lot and started to stretch my own adductors to see just how far I could get."

At this point our guide's head started to lower toward the floor, his legs going outward, and soon he too had assumed the not-possible-for-men position. Not only did our anatomy instructor accept his student's correction, but he embodied it in his own further inquiry, showing that humans can change perceptions and assumptions regarding the body, given the opportunity and flexibility of mind.

If we are taught in high school biology that the heart is a pump, this will be our primary metaphor for perceiving and evaluating the heart, perhaps including the implication of eventual mechanical failure. If we can expand our perceptions of our hearts, however, we can change how we live with them. The dominating metaphors for the heart that I learned were the structural, mechanical ones. I remember the drawings from high school and college biology with all the neat arrows to show blood flow. I recall sitting in a noontime conference with family practice residents and asking one about a valve. On

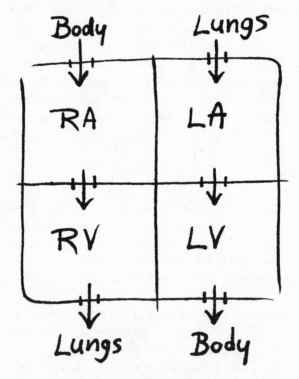

This "napkin schematic" of the heart, sketched by the physician who made this model both memorable and practical, shows the basic structures of the heart.

a napkin he hastily sketched out a box, which he subdivided into four boxes. He marked the valves and labeled the chambers all in the twinkling of an eye. This schematic drawing clarifies the parts, to be sure, but it ignores the organic and flexible curves of the heart and its capacity to function—to say nothing of the personal and cultural values we associate with it. The drawing reduces the heart to symmetrical, square chambers, a triumph of Cartesian abstraction, and the arrows show the direction of the flow of blood but give no hint to the amount of blood—which is to say the physiological efficiency. Traditionally, anatomy describes the *structures* of the heart, but physiology describes the *workings,* the function, the activity of the heart.

Both structure and function are important in the kind of heart surgery we'll see in the following story of Michael Kevin Curry. He came to Montana for repair of a sick heart: one valve had stopped working correctly. Because his heart no longer pumped blood properly, he became tired easily and could not live the active life of a man in his mid-twenties. He is, in fact, an athlete, and thus someone for whom physical activity is vitally important. Fortunately for him, cardiac assessment and surgery have both progressed to such levels of sophistication that his problem could be defined and fixed, albeit with some small risk. A generation or so back, he'd have been out of luck, doomed to a progressively weaker existence. In the course of Michael's story, a number of themes emerge—the search for understanding the heart's functions at a microscopic level, the significance of social support, the importance of patient attitude and motivation, and even an awareness of the spiritual dimensions—themes which will be elaborated on in the following sections of this book.

OFF AND ON THE CAROUSEL

The International Heart Institute of Montana is two floors above my office at St. Patrick Hospital in downtown Missoula. I take the stairs and meet Carole V. Erickson, who is administrative director of the institute; she has told me that the patient I'll be observing is Michael Kevin Curry, a twenty-seven-year-old athlete from Stanford, California. He's due in from the airport sometime around noon. I hang out in the lobby, fiddling with a jigsaw puzzle others have started. Good . . . most of the edge pieces have been sorted out. I link them up. I study the picture on the box. Garish sea creatures lurk below water; some heave themselves out of it. If I were a patient here or a family member, this would be a welcome diversion. Around 1:00 P.M. Carole brings a tall man over to me; he has black hair and a friendly smile. She introduces us. He calls me Dr. Carter, but I suggest Howard.

"Is it Michael or Mike?"

"Michael."

"Good. You had lunch?"

We walk out of the hospital and down a few streets to the Rhinoceros, a Missoula bar packed with animal heads, beer signs, and athletic trophies. There are fifty-nine colorful taps lining the bar, an inspiring sight. The news, however, is bad: the cook is on vacation for a month. So we walk down to the Stockman's Bar and Lunch (a common name in Montana towns) and sit at the bar. A menu on the wall in six-inch letters describes six kinds of hamburgers.

"Do you have bison burgers?" Michael asks.

"No, 'fraid not," the barkeep says.

"Moose Drool?" asks Michael, reading one of the six taps.

"Brewed right here. Dark beer. Very good."

"Heck, I gotta try that." We make jokes about the beer's logo, which shows large amounts of slobber dripping from a moose's snout. I recall a headline in a local paper, "Local Man Gored by Pet Elk."

I ask Michael about his running and triathlon career. For several years he competed in races. He had a very successful prep career. One man he competed with went on to the Olympics.

"You saw top action?"

"Yeah, I was part of it for a while."

"In college?"

"No . . . but like a lot of top high school runners, I was heavily recruited by several colleges. But I'm an all-or-nothing kind of guy. I knew I'd spend four, five hours a day training and a lot of other time worrying, strategizing, and so on. I went to Stanford because they paid absolutely no attention to my track experience."

"And did no athletics?"

"I rowed for a while. I guess I'm addicted to brutal endurance sports. Keeps you mellowed out."

"And now?"

"Heck, they won't let me lift weights: shoots up your blood pressure. At work we get a lot of old desks to fix up for the school; I shouldn't lift those either. I could run, but I don't like to because I can't go all out." He taps his chest over his heart.

From my modest career in the marathon and triathlon world, I know that athletes hate enforced rest.

Over the next few hours we move from the bar to the University of Montana campus. On the way we pick up his luggage from his motel. It's late September and the deciduous trees are just starting to turn. The grass is still green and lush. Students, walking by or riding by on their mountain bikes, are still wearing shorts and T-shirts. We visit a huge bronze statue of a grizzly bear (The Griz) in the center of a large quadrangle known as The Oval. We sit on the lawn and Michael tells me his story.

"Well, it all started from a cracked tooth . . . from a mint, right? I tell my friends, 'Be careful about hard candy—you might end up having heart surgery.'" We laugh. My laugh is a little strange because I'm eating a mint Michael has just offered from a small metal case.

"So I went to the dentist to get it fixed. And my mouth got all sore and red. It looked like strep, but the lab test came back negative. Anyway, I've had this great old doctor for years, African American, very kind, very calming, and he checked me all out. A wise soul, you know what I mean? I just had a low-grade fever, but he said my heart sounded a little odd and that I should come back in a week or so when the fever was gone. OK, so I did that, and the EKG showed some irregularities, which meant I got sent to a cardiologist.

"Well, the cardiologist did an echo—that's an echocardiogram—and saw that my aortic valve was leaking. He said, 'We can probably sit on that, just watch it for a while, but you have to be very careful about any dental work.' I said, 'Well, I just had dental work and my mouth was all sore and red.' So he gets this 'Oh, shit!' look on his face, and I know something's not good. They're supposed to hide that, aren't they? And he starts talking about sticking me in the hospital right away and stuffing antibiotic drugs into me through an IV. He pulls a bunch of heart valves out of his desk drawer and starts playing with them, spinning the little plastic disks and so forth, and says, 'If your heart valve is infected we may have to put one of these in you, and we may have to do it right away.' And that's all I remember, because I fainted and fell right out of my chair. The next thing I know six nurses were bringing me around.

"Now, I know I'm a bit of a hypochondriac—you know, like Woody Allen's character—the 'brain tumor' in *Annie Hall,* for example?—but the idea of heart surgery, being on blood thinners for the rest of your life—starting at age twenty-six—and the big-time antibiotics just freaked me out. And—get this—they said that my heart valve might be vegetating."

"Vegetating?" I say, trying to picture a little heart-valve garden, all varied shades of green, but no, Michael explained, the term indicates bacterial growth; certain bacteria and viruses love to live in the heart, and such vegetation can become so thick that it obstructs valve function.

"Well, despite the exciting possibility that my heart valve might be vegetating, it turned out—after another echocardiogram and some blood tests—that my heart was crying wolf. My heart murmur, this first time around, turned out to be mild, and the cardiologist thought that the antibiotics that had been given to me for possible strep throat had knocked out any minor heart infection as well." (I later learn that cardiologists don't consider any heart valve infection to be "minor," nor would a round of antibiotics for strep throat cure such a heart disease.)

"So the Woody Allen in you was disappointed?"

"You bet he was, but then came round two. A year and a half later I returned to Stanford to earn a master's in education, which meant that I had to change over to a new student health-care plan, which meant I had to obtain loads of referrals to get a checkup of my heart. I then met with a different cardiologist who said that maybe we could do an echo again, but maybe not. I was reluctant to do the test because the previous cardiologist had diagnosed my heart murmur as 'mild,' and I must say that in some sense I agreed with him, thinking at the time that another echo might be a waste of precious health-care dollars. But the Woody Allen in me won out, especially after I noticed that a cardiac resident standing behind the cardiologist was nodding his head up and down vigorously . . . so I asked him to order the echo so I wouldn't have to worry."

"And that's when you learned you had a real problem?"

"Yep . . . when this cardiologist returned with an analysis of the echo, he wore his own version of the 'oh, shit' look. He said that my ventricle had grown way beyond the upper end of normal. A year and a half before, during round one, it had been 5.7 cm, which was OK, given that I was 6'3" and a runner. My track coach—who was like a father to me—always said runners have big hearts. Right . . . but now mine's big—in the wrong way. I like to tell my friends—I work with impoverished kids while trying to fix up crummy schools—that I'm a bleeding heart liberal." For a moment I can hardly believe he's said that, but he's laughing and I'm laughing too.

"So that day—which was only a month or so ago—I learned that my left ventricle had swollen up to 7 cm in just eighteen months. And the valve, which had been leaking in the 'mild' range, is now called 'severe.' I'm just not getting enough blood out of that chamber, it's leaking back. The tapes . . ."

"What's that?"

"Oh yeah . . . I had to learn all this stuff . . . the ultrasound is put on tapes, you know like videotapes. I can carry them around so docs can review them. Some are in color, showing all the blood flow." I remember these from my Emory University observation; from a purely esthetic perspective, they're quite beautiful. (I described them in *First Cut* like this: "A computer process has colored the Doppler signals of the moving blood red, orange, and yellow, so that there are fluid explosions of dazzling color in the chambers and through the valves, a kind of liquid fireworks in the hypnotic rhythm of the beating heart.")

"And there's a sound." Michael imitates the *ski-wick, ski-wick* sound of pulsed blood flow; it sounds like a washing machine. "With a bass beat, even! I've got a friend who has epilepsy, and he's got some tapes from his neurology people. We've decided when we're both well we can give a party and mix our soundtracks for some totally funky effects." He pauses.

"So I went home and met with a surgeon friend of the family. He said the heart was swollen because of working 'uphill,' so to speak, but that it would return to normal size and function after surgery. My dad got real quiet . . . so I knew this was serious. But I didn't have any doubts about the decision: I needed work on my heart. The only question was when and where.

"One set of choices is total replacement with a mechanical valve—like the guy pulled out of his drawer, all those plastic and metals doodads that caused me to faint on the floor. Or you can get a pig valve. Or a homograft, you know, a valve from a human heart, probably from some guy who crashed his motorcycle. But all this isn't so hot for a young person, since you can develop troubles after fifteen to twenty years. For older people, that'd be cool; they say 'the repair will outlast the person.' Neat, huh? *The repair will outlast the person.*" He shakes his head, eyebrows raised. "But I'm twenty-seven. And then there's the other choice."

"What's that?"

"The Ross procedure—you've probably heard about it. They take out your aortic valve and throw it away, then move your pulmonary valve over to replace it. Obviously there can't be any rejection, because it's your own tissue, so you don't have to be on blood thinners forever. And then they stick in a sterilized homograft where your pulmonary valve was, and this does better there than in the aorta's place, because there's a lot less pressure. The heart pumps less hard for the short loop to the lungs than for the long loop to the rest of the body.

"Of course you want someone who's good at it, done it over forty times. Some docs start out and do OK for ten or twelve times but then have some complications. Some even give it up then. But the guys who stick it out get really good, and that's what I want."

"Makes sense to me."

"Besides, Arnold Schwarzenegger had the Ross . . . and he'll be right back in the pictures again. And Jesse Sapolu also had it, and he's still crushing quarterbacks for the 49ers," Michael says excitedly, smacking his fist into his open palm.

"Now the other thing that's tricky is the exact state of my valve. They even did a transesophageal echo. Basically they stick a probe down your gullet, and it sends out sound waves to the heart, so they get an even better look. Unfortunately echocardiograms and X-rays, and even just listening don't

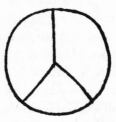

Sketch of a healthy closed aortic valve

produce exact results; in a way, doctors are still forced to play with shadows. They won't know exactly what's going on until they get in there. I'll have to give permission for both a valve repair and a Ross so they can decide once they get a direct look."

"What are the possibilities?"

"One is that the valve was congenitally deformed. Here, let me draw it for you." I hand Michael my pen and notepad. "The valve, if you look straight down at it, should look like a Mercedes Benz emblem, three leaflets all joining in the middle. When the blood pushes through, they open; then the blood pressure drops, because the ventricle relaxes, and they all go back together neatly—you know, a one-way valve—stopping any backflow. If they don't, the blood leaks back—get this, they call it 'regurgitation' [he makes a face], and the heart has to work harder to try to push it all out again."

"But then it could also be like this, a bicuspid valve, with two of the leaflets joined together in what they call a raphe." He draws, and I remember that the Greek root of raphe has to do with sewing; this anomaly would be the result of a variation in embryological development. "It did OK for twenty-seven years, but isn't as efficient as a regular tricuspid, and it is basically wearing out.

"Or this. . . ." He sketches. "Two of the leaflets have calcified and stuck to-gether—maybe from the infection of my dental work, maybe from something else. Who the hell knows? You gotta get in there and find out."

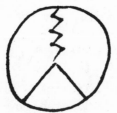 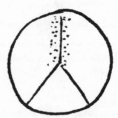

Sketches of a bicuspid valve with raphe (left) and a calcified tricuspid valve (right)

"Why here, then?"

"My dad's a retired CEO. He's used to solving problems . . . aggressively. We looked on the Web. We asked around. We remembered all the famous names. We picked ten places, and he wrote the same letter to all of them, outlining my case. We joked that they'd all want me because I'm a young athlete, the kind of patient that would improve their statistics.

"We got letters back, and Dr. Oury's was the one we liked best. He was straightforward and talked about the risks and longevity; he really spoke right to my situation. So we made some visits. Like picking a college, almost. One of the places we visited was like an assembly line. I was stuck in a maze of ropes like they have at the bank, you know, those velvet ropes on stands, with a bunch of eighty-year-olds. We were all clutching our paperwork and tickets, like at Disneyland, all in our hospital gowns. Then they decided somehow that I was a Peds [pediatric] patient, so they stuck me in with a bunch of kids. I had to sit on one of those stupid kindergarten chairs with my knees up around my ears.

"And we're on the phone with Montana . . . and everyone's nice and straightforward, so we had to come to this crazy little town and check it out.

"Doctor's offices—that's another thing. When I walk in, I want some signs of humanity. I've been in a lot of them now, and if they're business only or too dark, I kind of freeze up and know it's not right for me. Dr. Oury's office, though, has pictures of horses, his family, a climb he made up Mt. Kilimanjaro. I knew the minute I walked in he'd be a good guy to work with. The same goes for Dr. Hardy, too. He says he can hear a click of a bicuspid valve—so maybe that's what we've got.

"And that's about it." He stops and smiles.

"What happens next?"

"Well, I go home and give blood—for myself—over the next three, four weeks. It'll be stored then sent up here for my surgery. I've got to stop ten days before surgery and can only do a pint a week. On October 27 I fly back up, and they do a catheterization and explain everything to me again. The next day they operate and fix me up. Then it's five to seven days in the hospital. Then they want me to hang around for another week. Then I go home."

I've offered to drive Michael to the airport, all of ten minutes away, but his plane doesn't leave for another hour and a half.

"Do you like carousels?"

"Sure!"

Missoula's carousel is just a few years old, having opened in May of 1995. It was a community project, using the labor of hundreds of volunteers who worked for five years. It lies along the Clark Fork River in a park created by moving the river to the south. One of the first fully hand-carved carousels made in America since the Depression, it has a large and loud band organ and, of course, the colorful horses. My wife and I have visited the carousel several times, finding great joy in riding it, in seeing happy children and parents, in realizing that this is a focus for a healthy community.

"Do you understand about the rings?" I ask, pointing to a dragon figure alongside.

"Tell me."

"The dragon is loaded with a magazine of maybe fifty rings, all plastic except for the brass one, which gets you a free ride."

The carousel starts up and we watch children and adults whirl around, reaching out and up for the rings in the dragon's mouth.

"Oh, I get it. Of course, you have to be on the outside," Michael says.

"The competitive mind at work."

"Naturally."

"They list all the horses over here," I say, gesturing to a framed double-page spread from the local newspaper, the *Missoulian.*

Michael studies the horses with care and finds an Irish one. I'm Irish," he says. We've been talking about Butte, Montana, which had so many Irish miners that mail came from Ireland addressed directly to "Butte, America." I have an Irish-heritage woman from Butte in my class; she has white skin and black hair—like Michael. Michael frowns: "He'd better be on the outside, though."

We buy our tickets and ride the carousel. We grab plenty of plastic rings, but not the brass one. Afterward, Michael interviews the woman at the ticket booth, who informs us that the outside horses go eight-and-a-half miles per hour, making this one of the fastest carousels in the country. He buys a book about the Missoula carousel.

On our way to the airport, Michael says, "You know, all of this is going to work out great. I can see the signs. I was baptized at a St. Patrick's Church. My surgery's going to be at a St. Patrick Hospital. And now I ride on a horse covered with clovers and shamrocks. The carousel is kind of an image for life, right?—like at the end of *The Catcher in the Rye,* when Phoebe's going around and around, all vital and innocent. I'll come in October, have the surgery, and then jump back on the carousel."

Driving back from the airport, I muse over Michael's enthusiasm and commitment to his operation. His chest will be cut open, his heart stopped, and radical changes made. Would I be so sanguine about such things? Clearly he has faith in his surgeons, medical technology in general, and in the capacity of the body to heal from this dramatic intervention. He sees "signs," connections to aspects of his culture that give meaning and promise to his treatment, and he has created a story that forecasts a return to full activity, with no side effects, and does not include (as far as I know) the possibility of his death upon the operating table. If all goes well, he'll be the beneficiary of technology that is, quite literally, cutting edge.

STERILIZED HOMOGRAFTS AND OTHER WHOLEHEARTED EXPRESSIONS

Michael had to learn "all this stuff," and I'm following in his footsteps. I especially admire medical terms, which appear to have an exactitude, a rigorous precision. "Ejection fraction" means just that: the amount of blood expelled from the heart compared to the total amount in the left ventricle. The scientific English of articles in cardiac journals can be understood by adepts everywhere. "Sterilized homografts" mean just that, here in Montana or anywhere in the world. When I encounter terms I don't understand, I can find them in a medical dictionary or ask a medical person; the answers are always clear. These terms have a one-to-one (symbol-to-object) efficiency that rivals mathematics. They are fun to use because they give a feeling of being in charge. But I don't ordinarily find "ultrasound" or "catheterization" in poems. As a descriptive linguist might put it, scientific language is high in denotative value, giving a clear but sharply limited meaning with very little connotative value, the associative richness that poets love in, say, a word like "heart."

Michael enjoys language and has learned the scientific terms for his illness. But he also uses the more evocative words and phrases from everyday speech, such as "my heart was crying wolf." I enjoy talking with him because of his skill with language. As a writer, I'm obsessed with words in all their richness and readiness to combine in arresting and expressive ways. On a hunch that the English language may give some hints about our cultural heritage concerning hearts, I start a list of expressions that use some form of the word "heart." Before long I have over a hundred exhibits. I feel an urge to organize them, as a cowboy herds cattle into various pens. I know that some can go into more than one category, but—with the help of some dictionary listings—I find that five groups seem to work fairly well. I'll report on these throughout Michael's section. (Because of their multivalent meanings, some of them will repeat in later sections.)

The first group illustrates the *resolve* Michael and his parents displayed in assessing his need for medical care, not to mention the courage, a word with the Latin root of *cor,* or heart.

Here are the words and phrases: *strong-hearted, lionhearted, to be heartened, lighthearted, fainthearted, to lose heart, wholehearted, halfhearted, change of heart, his heart wasn't in it, break her heart, disheartened, brave heart, follow your heart's desire, I'd do it in a heartbeat, to have your heart in the right place, heart and soul, stirs the heart, take heart, heartily, with all your heart.*

Such words and phrases suggest the vitality we associate with the heart and the energizing of behavior through resolve, decisiveness, and steadiness of purpose. The Latin root *cor* gives us not only *courage* but also *cordiality* and *encouragement.* The liqueur called a *cordial* warms the *cockles of one's heart, cockle* deriving, according to one dictionary, from *cochlea,* or a winding cavern—therefore an innermost part. (The sensations of the stomach and the heart can be confused, owing to their common links to the cardiac plexus of nerves; a more serious confusion can occur when heartburn is interpreted as indigestion instead of a heart attack, thus delaying medical treatment.)

According to this group of words, the heart is a dynamo, a ticker, a main-spring, a powerhouse, the home of *élan vital,* drive, or, simply, power that mo-tivates humans to do whatever they choose, even including having their chests cut open for cardiac surgery. Many of these phrases are positive, but to act *in a heartbeat* may be a reckless, ill-considered choice. Or it could be a generous act to a friend. Following *your heart's desire* may be narcissistic. Having *your heart in the right place* is tautologically good, and, in general, it is good (in this culture) to be *wholehearted* and not namby-pamby or wishy-washy. Such values seem particularly western: questing, striving, searching. Richard the Lionhearted was a crusader, saving the Holy Land from, presumably, the non-lionhearted. By contrast, some of Henry James's stories present characters who lacked heart, as in "The Beast in the Jungle": poor John Marcher (the last name is ironic) has plodded through life never accepting the call of his heart.

In this set of meanings, the heart may be defined as a wellspring and a home for courage and resolve, or, in expressions such as *fainthearted,* a lack of such qualities.

Cardiac Holy Grails

Carlos M. G. Duran, M.D., Ph.D., is President and CEO of the International Heart Institute of Montana. He and his colleagues have hosted an annual conference in Missoula for some twenty years: cardiologists from all over the world come to hear the latest news, watch surgery, and practice techniques on the fully cooperative hearts that have come from pigs. Duran's specialty is heart valves; he's the inventor of the Duran Ring, a device used to stabilize replaced valves. A cabinet in the lobby displays a series of bioengineered heart valves, some large, some small, made up of a variety of materials: metal, ceramic, plastic, and substances I don't recognize. A Spaniard by origin, Dr. Duran has studied in England and France. "Do you know why they call it the 'morgue?'" he asks me. "Because the original place for cadavers in Paris was on the Rue Morgue—which also shows up in the Poe short story."

His office walls display some of Leonardo da Vinci's Windsor drawings of the heart. "These are surprisingly useful," he says, gesturing to a framed drawing, "although no one had any idea of his accuracy for centuries. Leonardo shows the valves in wonderful detail and gives a good idea of the swirls and whorls of blood flow within the heart." *Swirls and whorls,* I think, not the linear flow of the Cartesian boxes.

We sit at a table, and he continues. "We like cryopreserved valves. They are taken from cadavers, trimmed, maintained in antibiotics, and cooled down to -180° C. They have to be transported in liquid nitrogen and stored in special refrigerators. A team of nurses must be specifically trained not only to handle the cryopreserved valve but also to obtain the donor hearts. All these conditions represent a considerable commitment of the hospital and of the cardiac team. The main problem is the very limited availability of good, young donor hearts. Although these valves would be an ideal solution to the millions of patients that need a new aortic valve in the developing world, the complexity of the process makes impossible its clinical application. Even in the United States they're hard to transport, and a blackout can put you out of business: if they warm up at the wrong time, you can't use them." These are called "homografts," meaning grafts from the same species (humans). Heterografts would be from another species, such as pigs. For years, pig valves have been used in humans; a Jewish friend of mine received one years ago. He thought it was ironic, even hilarious, but also justified by a Talmudic teaching that advocated the primacy of saving life.

Dr. Duran continues, "What you want is the collagen matrix for a scaffold over which a person's own cells will grow. Cells are funny creatures . . . they do what the hell they want. You have to trick them into growing in the right places." He goes on to talk rapidly about myocytes, cardiac geometry, fourth-power radii, and things I can't really follow. What I do get is that he's a man in love with hearts in all their aspects, a disciple of Heart. He's interested in the application of all the tricks western biomedicine can bring to the heart's structural and cellular nature. The Batista operation, for example, is based on the surgical reduction in the diameter of the much dilated heart by simply cutting a large slice of muscle. Duran likes the boldness of the idea but doesn't think it has proved itself yet. He's more interested in a series of laser points burned into the heart muscle so that the heart can revascularize and become more healthy. But most of all he's involved with the Ross procedure, one of the institute's specialties. Donald Ross, an English surgeon, developed the procedure in 1967 to replace a failing aortic valve. It's now done around the world, and the institute maintains a registry for the technique's results and follow-ups. The operation was first done in the United States in 1991; as of my observation, over twelve hundred have been done, with statistically very good results in terms of patient survival, the lack of need for revision (a second operation), and the heart's performance in pumping blood—*hemodynamics,* in the technical terminology.

"This is the best time to be in medicine," Dr. Duran says excitedly. "We're just at the brink of discoveries that will change cardiology radically." I think of all the complaints about medicine: HMO and insurance controls, legal risks, bioethical dilemmas, expense, maldistribution of doctors (rural vs. urban), the aging population, the lack of preventive medicine—a constellation of factors that has sent some doctors out of the profession and has discouraged some people from entering it. But he continues, "I think that it will be bigger than the information revolution. I am thinking of Angiogenesis or the development of new vessels and of the impact of the statins not only as a cholesterol-reducing drug but also their anti-inflammatory properties. We now know the tremendous role of inflammation in the development of coronary plaques.

"And take tissue engineering. I'll have you meet Dr. Cheung and Dr. Pang upstairs. They're working on the cellular level of hearts and finding wonderful things. If all goes well, we'll find the Holy Grail of valves, a living valve that will renew itself, with no chance of rejection, with no need for future surgical revision, and with an unlimited time horizon. The best we can do now is to give a patient one of his own valves through the Ross procedure."

We walk down the hall and up the back stairs to the labs above. On a lab bench is an oversize model of the heart, about two fists' worth. "This is the Torrent-Guasp model," Dr. Duran says, unfolding the red, rubbery thing. It's a shell within a shell that unwinds to about two feet long. "Dr. Torrent thinks the myocardium is best understood as four units that wrap like this." He twirls the irregular strip back into a compact heart. "This is so exciting, a whole new way of conceptualizing the heart—that it's one long band of muscle. This goes against standard teachings today, even the embryonic understanding, but it answers some questions and gives some insights for surgery. We need challenges to keep us thinking. Still, it's not yet the whole story. I've got some ideas myself, but I'm still learning. At this point I'm wrong . . . but maybe less wrong than other theorists."

Dr. Duran introduces me to David Cheung, Ph.D., a collagen chemist. Dr. Cheung explains to me the biochemistry of sterilized valves, how they're taken from a cadaver, chemically stripped of cells that might cause compatibility problems, and trimmed so that they can be put into live hearts. He shows me little vials containing tan rings—the collagen armature—a dry, sterilized valve ready for a new home. Without any fluid surrounding it, it weighs almost nothing, little more than the plastic container resting in my hand. The goal is to make such a valve attractive to the host's own living cells that will colonize this matrix. "It's got to be a *living* cell," he says with passion. "Everyone has been talking about valves being biocompatible, but now it's time to talk about them being biointegratable. What's next? Bio"—he searches for a word "bio*active,* as we create valves that can travel all over the world, with no refrigeration, no chemical bath, but ready to *live* in a new body. And we could move on to other implants as well, cartilage, blood vessels, entire organs . . . who knows where this will end?"

Dr. Cheung shows me slides of various kinds of cardiac tissue. As we leave the lab to go into his office, we pause at a set of photographs taped to his door. These were taken through a microscope, evidently from very thin tissue slices that have been stained, causing the thin cell walls and the nuclei to stand out clearly. "What's this?" I ask.

"Cardiac scar tissue. How do the cells lie?"

I look at the chaotic swirls. "They're all jumbled up."

"Exactly. It's a real mess. We've got to figure out why and help them reform into proper layers."

Dr. Cheung hands me off to David Pang, Ph.D., a biologist. I'm not sure how much more my brain can absorb, but Dr. Pang takes off like a rocket, leading me to a computer, where he puts in a CD. Little Xs show up on the screen and pulsate rhythmically. "A heart?" I guess.

"It's a sheep's heart." He turns a control and slows down the rhythm. He points to an X. "Each point is a piezoelectric crystal that we've placed in the tissues. The crystals function as miniature transducers, sending out mini pulses, so small that they don't interfere with each other. Like this one here." He holds up a thin wire with a tiny crystal at the end, so small I can barely see it. "We call this sonomicrometry—a kind of ultrasound. We collect the impulses and feed them to the computer which creates this array." He works the controls, speeding up then slowing down the dancing points. He slows them down to a crawl. "With this technique we can find hidden movements of the heart. Look right here. This is the aorta, which is about to receive blood from the ventricle." I see a set of points that define a space—or, more accurately, suggest a volume. He turns the controls and they separate from each other slightly. He adjust his glasses and smiles, "That's great . . . we've found that the aortic root expands just *before* the valve opens."

"And the same would be true in humans?"

"We don't know yet, but we think so. See what this *means?*" he says, smacking the desk top. "The heart isn't just a force pump pushing blood on through . . .

it's also a *suction* pump—even beyond the last valve—*pulling* the blood at the same time. And that's a whole new concept in how the heart works."

Aha . . . so it's not just a force pump, hammering blood through mechanical spaces, but rather an organic set of malleable chambers. And perhaps it can pull as well as push, and certainly it is an organ with its own genius, including many secrets within its many cells, secrets still to be discovered and described.

ESSENCE, CENTER

I'm dazzled by the research of Dr. Duran and his colleagues, not simply because of the different models and imaginative thought, but because of the motivation, the drive to find, in his words, the "Holy Grail of valves," and all other innermost secrets of the heart's organization and capacities—the heart of the heart, so to speak. (William H. Gass's story "In the Heart of the Heart of the Country" comes to mind.) Indeed we use heart language to speak of the essential qualities of something, the deepest, most central qualities.

I've collected the following: *the heart of a city, the heart of the problem, at heart, heartland of America, heart of the matter, deep in the heart of Texas, home is where the heart is, heart of stone, heart of gold* (and *whore with a heart of gold*), *cut the heart out of, stab in the heart, strike to the heart, heartwood, kindhearted, young at heart, after my own heart, lay to heart.*

Such expressions suggest the innermost nature of something, its hidden essence. The word *essence* is built from the Latin *esse, to be;* what is the fundamental being of the heart? How does it exist? How may this be determined? Heart researchers want to know and try a variety of approaches. A doctor treating a patient for heart ailment wants to understand the problem. A heart patient wants a diagnosis and treatment so that she or he can resume an active life. Persons interested in their health want to know how the heart works and how it may be cared for. For some, perhaps, the heart is out of sight and, therefore, out of mind.

What is the basic essence of anything (the focus of ontology), and how may we know it (the focus of epistemology)? Our language suggests that the heart, the vital organ that makes our lives possible, is a good metaphor for central qualities—which may not be readily apparent. The literary cliché of the "whore with a heart of gold" promises an inner value not apparent from outward appearance or behavior. We generally know that our hearts are necessary for our biological lives, but how often do we find the heart of a community, a city, or our country? Politicians claim to know the heart of the electorate, and they love to visit the heartland of America (however defined), but we know that they often speak to the middle of a bell-shaped curve created by focus groups, polls, and advisers—a statistical, tactical "heart" of persons likely to vote or donate money.

Drs. Duran, Hardy, and Oury follow some two millennia of thinkers and researchers who want to know the essence of the physiological heart. The essential nature of a patient such as Michael depends on such knowledge and its careful application.

MEDICINE AND THE HEART

The medical understanding of the heart that makes Michael's operation not only possible but even routine was a long time coming. Modern cardiology is a scant generation or two old now, even though medical interest in the heart goes back to ancient times. Given the heart's centrality in the body, and its obvious pulses that suggest life and death, probably most cultures took some technical interest in its structure and function. The ancient Chinese, for example, used charts of pulses at the wrist to assess the health of the heart; one appears in *Secrets of the Pulse,* dating from the sixth or fifth century B.C.E. The following discussion will, however, focus on western medicine.

By the time of Aristotle, in the fourth century B.C.E., the heart was considered the site of consciousness. In *Parts of Animals* (humans included), Aristotle gives detailed descriptions of the structure of the heart, although his sense of physiology is, by modern standards, vague and inexact. He felt that the brain somehow radiated heat, while the heart produced and maintained heat for the body. In the heart he discerned three cavities, each filled with blood. He saw connections to the lungs, and assumed that the heart mixed air and blood. The heart was the center of sensation. According to Lyons and Petrucelli (*Medicine: An Illustrated History,* [New York: Harry N. Abrams], 1978), Aristotle linked veins from the liver to the right arm and veins from the spleen to the left arm; since he also had some faith in the four-humour theory (blood, black bile, yellow bile, and phlegm), he felt that bloodletting should, therefore, be on the same side of the body as the diseased organ. Aristotle, and later Galen, were immensely influential right up to the Renaissance. (Humours are the source of our modern sense of "humor": a humorous person was originally a person with one humour so prominent as to be worthy of satire and laughter.)

In the second century C.E., Galen wrote several treatises on the pulse; he felt that regularity, strength, and speed were all diagnostic of a patient's health. His anatomical experience was limited to animals and wounded gladiators, however, and he described aspects of the heart that were not accurate, for example, pores between the right and left heart that would allow blood to seep through. His assumption of these pores—he admitted they were hard to see—was a necessity of his theory, according to Jonathan Miller (*The Body in Question* [New York: Random House, 1978]). Galen also drew on the four-element theory (and the corresponding humours) and the vitalist principle—also called *pneuma* or *thymos*—which he called "Natural Spirits." Although he may have had enough information to see the heart as a pump, Miller suggests, he did not have the surrounding technological culture of pumps to give him this metaphor. Instead, he saw the heart as a kind of lamp or furnace that regulated hot and cold, mixed blood and breath. Galen's influence was enormous and long-lasting—some twelve hundred years. During this time, his authority—at least in the West—was taken as absolute. Indeed, it was said that if a body structure did not conform to Galen, it was an error of nature.

The Middle Ages made little progress in anatomy, owing in part to strictures from the church against cutting up the dead. Four-element theories continued (still a justification for bloodletting), joined by alchemy and even astrology, which suggested a correspondence between—not surprisingly—the heart and the sun sign Leo, as in our phrase "lionhearted." More specifically, the alchemists saw the heart as an image of the sun within man, parallel to gold, the image of the sun on (or in) earth. A 1522 woodcut shows a man standing erect with the twelve zodiacal emblems superimposed upon his body, just twenty years before the work of Andreas Vesalius changed dramatically medicine's perception of the body.

With the Renaissance, perceptions of the heart began to change in the direction toward modern thinking. Andreas Vesalius published his *De humani corporis fabrica* (*The Fabric of the Human Body;* 1543), based on his extensive dissection of human bodies. While Vesalius made many respectful references to Galen, he also disagreed with him at points, for example, the interseptal holes in the heart Galen had described but that Vesalius could not find. In mentioning Galen's lack of direct experience with human cadavers ("he himself never dissected the body of a man who had recently died"), Vesalius sets a new standard for scientific truth, the empirical method: researchers should do their own experiments in great detail and not rely on the authority of predecessors. This is a Renaissance breakthrough, the inductive approach that still holds in experimental science in general and in medicine in particular. Old and new views of the heart are constantly held up to scrutiny to see if they are adequate.

Also important are the detailed woodcuts of *De humani corporis fabrica*, many of which are still reprinted today because of their clarity and beauty. The dissected figures are covered with Greek and Roman letters corresponding to Vesalius's identifications in the text. These illustrations—like the drawings of

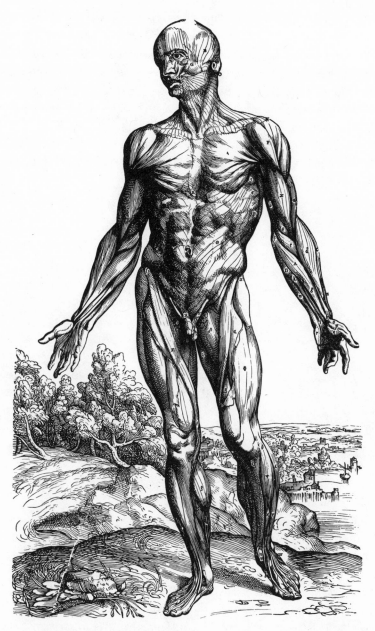

A "muscle man" woodcut from Andreas Vesalius. Vesalius published the first comprehensive anatomy book based on direct and minute observation of cadavers. The Latin title *De humani corporis fabrica* (1543) may be translated as "Concerning the fabric of the human body." The illustrations are famous for their accuracy and detail. One set has figures standing in landscapes as if alive, although their skin and subdermal fat have been removed to show the outermost muscles clearly.

da Vinci (those admired by Dr. Duran) to come in another sixty years or so and the engravings of *Gray's Anatomy* in the late nineteenth century—set a new standard in modeling physical structures accurately and clearly. Medicine rests on such observation and representation; in the case of hearts, especially, varying modalities have made more and more sophisticated diagnostic tools and treatments possible: the stethoscope, X-rays, EKGs, echosonography, CT scans, MRIs, and nuclear medicine.

Vesalius, however, equivocates about the sorts of animal spirits the ancients spoke of, *pneuma* or *thymos*. He speaks in his preface of the heart as "the tinder

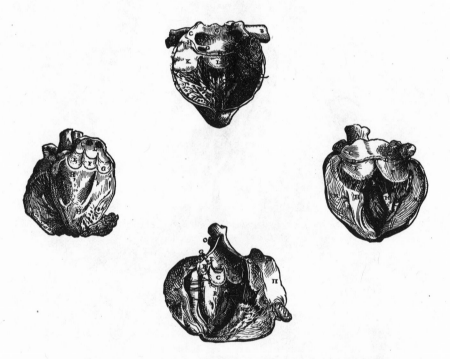

Four views of the heart from Vesalius's *De humani corporis fabrica*. Vesalius, who, like Galen, believed that there was an ebb and flow motion of blood, did not understand circulation. In the ancient view the heart was a two-chambered organ, requiring blood to "sweat" through the interventricular septum. Vesalius, however, based on his direct observation of the heart, began to doubt this explanation. It was only with William Harvey's studies roughly a century later that the circulation was considered circular throughout the body. That there are four views here is suggestive; the perceived nature of the heart depends on the point of view (including assumptions, values, learning, and behavior) of the perceiver.

of the vital faculty," but his emphasis in some seven hundred pages that follow is on structure, not religion or natural philosophy. With Vesalius, modern
anatomy is born and, some have said, modern medicine. The heart is now a
discrete set of tissues, like the muscles of the leg, that can be taken apart and
studied in elaborate detail. (Indeed, it may be said that the drawings are so
clear as to be misleading; students opening a cadaver will find an interwebbed
chaos of many colors, not the black-and-white, schematic clarity of Vesalius.) Finally, the engravings of *De humani corporis fabrica* are not neutrally
objective. Echoing Renaissance graphics and classical sculpture, they show
complexity of the body with its own stature and magnificence. Supernatural
forces or gods are not needed to animate these cadavers; they have their own
humanistic glory.

The second great figure of the Renaissance to change perceptions of the
heart was the Englishman William Harvey. While forerunners (Servetus,
Columbo, Cesalpino) had suggested a circulation of blood throughout the
body, Harvey wrote the book that established the concept of the heart as a
pump, using his practical methods of analysis and elegant reasoning. *De motu
cordis et sanguinis* (*On the Motion of the Heart and Blood*) was published in
1628 and went through many editions. Harvey used a focused approach; as
Lyons and Petrucelli put it, "he concerned himself solely with the mechanical
flow of blood, not with what happened in the heart, liver, and brain." Harvey
understood the heart as a pump—not a lamp, not a locus for emotions or
thought—that sent blood around the body. He couldn't see the capillary link
between the arterial system and the venous system, but he had faith that it
was there. Only with the invention of the microscope could Marcello Malpighi
establish the existence of capillaries. Harvey lived in the emerging industrial
age, which may have supplied him with his basic image for the heart, a force
pump, but he also felt an Aristotelian influence in that he saw the circular motion of the blood around the body as an echo of universal circularities, such as
rain and evaporation, even "tempests and meteors." The trend toward modern
medicine, of course, has been to strip away abstract universalities, Natural
Spirits, resonances with astrology, the heavens, the gods. René Descartes,
often invoked as the conceptual father of the modern computer, did his best
to separate ideas and materials, even within the human form, a dualism or
split of mind and body. In his *Discourse on Method* (1637) Descartes referred
to Harvey's work, supposing that it represented the mechanical absolutes of
the body. While the god-given soul was different from such slings and levers
of the body, Descartes believed that warmth was central to the activity of the
heart and that breathing somehow directly fueled "the fire of the heart." His
mixture of vitalism and mechanism kept the mind, the soul, and the brain

separate from bodies, however, so that animals and humans were—at the level of the body—basically the same. The scientific approach (from Francis Bacon and others) favored direct observation, cause-and-effect reasoning, scientific instrumentation, and measurement in numbers. These traits accorded well with industrialization, engineering, and the mechanical metaphors that reshaped, in part, our view of the human body. The invention of the "pulse watch" (a watch with a second hand) in 1707 by John Floyer was an invention we now take for granted. This instrument allowed for the first time the quantification of pulses, one of the five vital signs routinely taken today. For Dr. Floyer—who had read Galen on pulses—the heart was to be regulated like a machine: "The Physicians' Business is to regulate the Circulation, and to keep it in a moderate degree . . . if it run oftner or slower, our Mechanism is out of order." By applications of heat and cold, Floyer felt he could treat disease and, therefore, the heart. He believed "our Senses can sufficiently inform us of all the most useful PHOENOMENA whereby we know or cure our Diseases, or prognosticate concerning them."

In broad terms, the reshaping of the modern medical view of the heart brought by Vesalius and Harvey has several implications. The ancient Natural Spirits and circular perfections of the Greeks are gone; even the Christian notion of the home of the soul was left aside. The heart's meaning has been redefined as a durable pump with an important job. Medicine's job (a version of Dr. Floyer's pronouncement) is to keep the pump running as long and as efficiently as possible.

Our most common instrument for perceiving the heart, the stethoscope, originated with Parisian physician René Laennec early in the nineteenth century. The story goes that two children playing with a wooden board invited him to hear the scratchings of a pin being transmitted down its length. Inspired, Laennec tried a rolled-up sheaf of papers and then a wooden tube to listen to his patients' hearts as never before.

The word "stethoscope" is made up of the Greek roots for *chest* and *seeing,* although *perceiving* would be a more accurate translation in this case. Previously, male physicians had placed their heads on the chests of patients; the new device avoided that awkwardness with women patients. A relatively simple device, an inexpensive stethoscope can now be purchased at a medical supply store for about ten dollars. Miniaturized echocardiography machines may replace stethoscopes in some offices and clinics; these are about the size of a laptop and can do an exam in eight minutes, as opposed to twenty minutes on the full-sized model. Their price (currently twelve thousand dollars) will, however, keep the regular stethoscope in business.

The electrocardiogram, another technological mainstay for heart care, was developed at the end of the nineteenth century. While various scientists had looked at electrical impulses in the body, it was the Dutch physician Willem Einthoven who figured out a sensitive but reliable method of measuring electrical activity in the heart. He refined the device and the techniques for its use over the course of thirty years, winning the Nobel Prize for physiology/medicine in 1924. (While some Americans use ECG for electrocardiogram, we commonly see EKG for electrokardiogram, the German parallel, indicating the origin of its manufacture.) The twelve-lead EKG is common today: twelve electrodes gather electrical news, which is amplified and converted into a series of graphs displayed on a monitor or printed onto slips of paper. (We'll see this machine in action later.)

In the history of humanity, cardiac surgery is a very recent development. By the end of the nineteenth century, modern anesthesia made surgery in many areas of the body possible, but surgeons still left the heart alone. Theodor Billroth and Stephen Paget spoke out against heart surgery of any kind: they felt that the heart was naturally too difficult to work with and that surgeons should respect this limit. According to medical journalist Lawrence K. Altman, "As late as the 1920s . . . it was taboo for a doctor to touch the living human heart." In 1929, however, Werner Forsmann ran a urethral catheter up a vein in his arm and into his heart to measure the pressure of the right ventricle. By doing so, he made possible, in concept, many of the diagnostic tests and procedures we have today. The heart was no longer inviolable; it was a wonderfully complex organ that could be not only touched but also worked on. With the introduction of heart-lung machines in the 1950s, still more became possible, as patients' hearts could be operated on without blood flowing through them, making possible valve repairs, the Ross procedure, and transplantation. Beyond the strictly surgical techniques, the medical approach saw increasing sophistication in cardiac drugs. And epidemiology, behavioral medicine (stress studies), and genetics (family history) have added further perspectives. With advances in minimally invasive surgery (through catheters—small tubes instead of large, open wounds), analysis of the human genome, and the biochemical study of cardiac tissue (as in the Heart Institute's lab), further resources will be available to both doctors and their patients.

Dr. Oury, Dr. Duran, Dr. Hardy, and many other cardiac surgeons have the abilities, the equipment, and the courage to repair a heart, to fix it up *as good as new;* such news allows me to feel that there is a back wall, a safety net, a structural backup for our hearts. Nonetheless, many other things can go wrong with the heart, can go wrong with machines, can go wrong in hospitals. The risks are omnipresent in sickness and in health—we just don't like to think about them. And I also know that most of the world's population can't afford cardiac surgeries.

Furthermore, there have been two profound losses in our relationship to our hearts. First, the biomedical models have become so arcane that we have given up knowing our hearts in any detail beyond the general notion that it is a pump and that we should, in general, take care of it. Second, we have, by and large, lost various notions of the ancients that ennobled the heart: that it was the home for the soul; that it was a lamp or furnace, a hearth of sorts that kept us going; that it was the home for thinking and feeling; that it was a meeting place with the divine. In the modern view, only thinking found a new home, in the brain. The other qualities were disenfranchised, kicked out of the heart, sent into exile—at least in the scientific view. Popular culture and artists (the romantics, in particular), however, have kept the cultural sense of the heart alive. The surgery that will be used in the attempt to repair Michael's heart was founded on knowledge of wonderful sophistication, but Michael didn't select his doctors for their technical knowledge alone. Other aspects of their humanity, such as the items in Dr. Oury's office, were signals to him that Missoula offered the best chance for the healing of his heart.

WHICH IS DEEPER, KNOWLEDGE OR WISDOM?

The heart, like many subjects of study, acts as a mirror of the researchers: the heart reflects the assumptions and methods of a given age or, with modern acceleration, of a generation or less. Knowledge evolves through various paradigms; scientific investigation finds new tools, such as echosonography. Because Aristotle subscribed to the humour theory, he saw the physiology of the heart acting in a congruent way. After the industrial revolution, the heart was interpreted mechanically, measurable by a watch. Nonscientists such as the Romantics, however, maintained the tradition that the heart was a repository—at least symbolically—of insight, intuition, and deep knowledge, a tradition that goes back to biblical times. While our modern consciousness understands the concepts of blood pressure and pulse, and of the mechanical nature of a blocked coronary artery, we persist in using phrases that suggest that the heart is a place of wisdom, even though we give primacy to the brain as the place of reason and memory.

Consider the following phrases in our language: *I know in my heart, to ponder something in my heart, in my heart of hearts, lay to my heart, take to heart, winning hearts and minds, after my own heart, I know that song by heart.* These phrases suggest that the heart is the repository for things we know, from the relatively simple memorization of a song or text to a depth knowledge that partakes of mystical intuition. This kind of knowing is different from (and perhaps deeper than) mere knowledge of facts; it may include kinds of understanding that we don't yet have names for. To indicate a deep thought, conviction, or feeling, we sometimes touch our chest.

In the book of Sirach, wisdom is a woman named Sophia. Today we speak of a woman's intuition. In the book of Luke, "Mary pondered these things in her heart." Women's wisdom has been less in fashion during periods dominated by enlightenment and scientific thought, although there's been a renaissance through contemporary women's studies, the work of Carol Gilligan, for example. Male-dominated education promotes mathematical-based science, not courses in intuition. Outside of academia, there were the hippies' "bad vibrations, man," a gut (heart?) sense that someone or some place was not good.

Michael understands the basic biology and physics of his failing heart and the proposed repair; he has faith in contemporary cardiology. He also senses the character of Dr. Oury through the decor of his office, clues to another kind of knowledge that Michael finds comforting.

THE PUMP

The common contemporary view of the heart is that it is a pump, and one worth caring for. Indeed, Americans in the last twenty years have become more heart conscious; the mass media trumpets much about diet, exercise, smoking cessation, and stress reduction. Some restaurants print hearts by the low-fat dishes in their menus. Burger stands now have salads; some even offer veggie burgers. And heart disease has diminished somewhat, although not equally across all economic classes of Americans. African Americans, for example, are more prone to high blood pressure, a principal cause of heart disease.

The standard teaching of western biology and medicine understands the heart as a functioning structure. The human heart has four chambers, two atria stacked on top of two ventricles. Each atrium, like the atrium of an office building, is an entryway, in this case to the larger ventricle below it. "Ventricle," at its root, means "little belly," a small volume that can be expanded by the blood we "feed" into it. If the oxygen from the lungs may be considered a food of a sort, carrying the oxygen in blood through our bodies, the heart, in sending oxygenated blood throughout the body, does indeed nourish us. (Anyone who has been anemic, that is, low in the red blood cells that carry oxygen, knows the weakness of such malnourishment.) The heart itself resides at the midline of the chest and extends to the left. (In the description that follows, *left* and *right* refer, in the tradition of anatomy, to the orientation of the body studied and

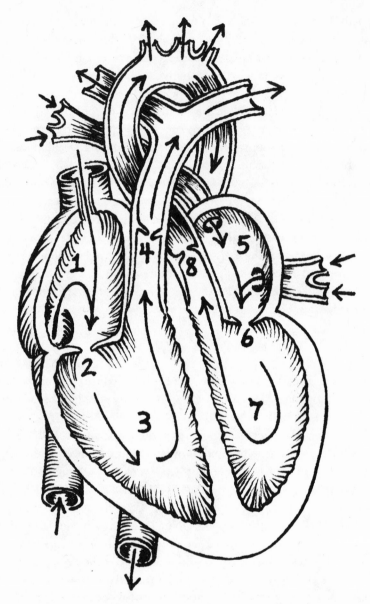

This drawing of the four-chambered heart is based on standard renderings in anatomy-physiology texts for college students. The basic structural components follow the pump metaphor of how the heart works in receiving blood from the body (1. right atrium, 2. tricuspid valve), sending it to the lungs (3. right ventricle, 4. pulmonary valve), then receiving it, oxygenated, from the lungs (5. left atrium, 6. mitral valve), and sending it back out to the body (7. left ventricle, 8. aortic valve). In Michael's surgery, the failing aortic valve (8.) is replaced by his pulmonary valve (4.), which is replaced by a sterilized valve from a cadaver.

not to the observer's point of view.) There are individual variations, however, and some predictable relocations; for example, in late pregnancy, the expectant mother's heart is pushed up and to her left. In cases of situs inversus, all the internal organs, the heart included, are on the opposite side from normal.

The right atrium receives venous blood from the body, low in oxygen, high in carbon dioxide; blood donors can see this dark, brownish-red blood slowly filling the plastic bag. When the right atrium contracts, the venous blood is pushed downward through the tricuspid valve and into the right ventricle. When the lower heart contracts, the blood is propelled through the pulmonary valve toward the lungs. The valves are like doors for restaurant kitchens: they open only in one direction to keep traffic orderly. In the lungs the necessary gas exchanges (carbon dioxide out, oxygen in) occur on the surface of the red blood cells, before the blood returns to the heart with the bright red color we usually think of for blood. Returning via the pulmonary veins to the left atrium, it is then pumped downward through the mitral valve to the left ventricle. Finally, the left ventricle, with its strong thick walls, contracts and shoots blood up through the aortic valve and into the elegantly curved aorta on its way to the entire body. From the aorta, the coronary arteries immediately branch off, turning right back to the heart itself to give the oxygen necessary for this continuously working muscle. If a coronary artery is blocked, insufficient oxygen reaches cardiac tissue, and the tissue dies: a heart attack, or, in doctor talk, a myocardial infarction. (*Myo* means muscle, *cardio* means heart, *infarction* means necrosis or tissue death caused by a blockage; "MI" is the oft-heard abbreviation.)

The carotid arteries sprout upward from the aorta to service the head (especially the brain, a big user of oxygen); continuing on down the descending aorta, we find arteries branching off to serve our internal organs, our musculature, our skin—in sum, the entire body. The circulatory system serves directly almost every cell of the body, excluding only the cornea of the eye and the outermost layer of skin; by one estimate there are sixty thousand miles of blood vessels in a human. The so-called white tissues of ligament and cartilage are sparsely supplied with blood, one reason injuries to them can take a long time to heal. Besides transporting gases, the blood stream (including the allied lymphatic system) absorbs nutrients from digested food in the small intestine and distributes them around the body. Blood passes through the liver for chemical regulation, passes through the kidneys for the withdrawal of waste, and transports hormones from the ten endocrine glands to various target tissues all around the body. Thus the bloodstream is the internal transportation system of the body, with several main branches and many, many progressively finer vessels. Block this fine plumbing (with a blood clot or a large plaque, say), and the starved cells downstream become dysfunctional and die.

In the hydraulic terms of the pump metaphor, the pressure generated at the wellhead of the heart slowly falls as the blood meets resistance throughout the body. A nurse taking our blood pressure with a cuff on the upper arm measures the two pressures in the brachial artery as a wave of blood pulses through. The resulting numbers represent the height of mercury in a glass tube (expressed as millimeters of mercury, symbolized as Hg); this height implies a corresponding weight, which approximates the pressure in an artery. In earlier days, such a column was mounted on the wall. In contemporary instruments—and especially in portable ones—a dial or digital numbers give a comparable readout. For a typically healthy reading of 120/80 mm/Hg ("one-twenty over eighty"), the upper number represents the pressure wave from the heart, or the systolic pressure. (Systole means contraction of the heart.) The lower number represents the constant pressure between beats of the heart, or the diastolic (*dia* means *across* or *through,* as in *diameter*); this pressure is the same as the resistance offered by the arteriolar walls, the pressure against which the heart must pump. Both numbers are important measures of the health of the system and any changes in it. A person whose cardiovascular system is opened, so that they lose large amounts of blood—externally or internally—will obviously lose blood pressure. The heart, stimulated by a feedback loop, will pump faster, trying to make up the difference. For the paramedic, a pulse rising above 100 bpm (beats per minute) and a systolic pressure falling below 100 mm/Hg represents an approximate sign that a patient is going into shock. The pump is trying to get the blood through the vascular system (including its own cardiac arteries), which is failing for one or more reasons: neurological messages to shut down capillaries, damage to the heart itself, or loss of blood. If you open the system up enough, a person can bleed to death in about two minutes. One definition of shock is simply "inadequate tissue perfusion," which means the pump is not getting blood around to service the entire organism. At some point circulation to the brain will be inadequate, and the person will lose consciousness. If the brain is without oxygen (a condition called anoxia) for three minutes or more, damage is likely. Within another few minutes, the person dies.

The two upper chambers, the atria, contract together, sending blood to the ventricles. When their valves (the tricuspid and the mitral) close approximately at the same time, the two other valves (the aortic and pulmonary) open up at approximately the same time; the resulting noise is what we hear as the first heart sound. When the two lower chambers, the ventricles, contract together, they send blood on the short loop to the lungs and on the long loop to the body. When their parallel valves (the pulmonary, sending blood from the heart to the lungs, and the aortic, sending blood through the aorta to the rest of the body) close, and the tricuspid and the mitral open, the resultant noise is the second heart sound. If we see a beating heart during an operation, the upper and lower chambers alternate in swelling and emptying in parallel fashion—high, low, high, low—in a hypnotic rhythm. It looks graceful, even easy, but, in fact, heart muscles work hard. A common museum demonstration is a mounted tennis ball; visitors are asked to squeeze it with one hand to approximate the force needed to contract the heart and expel a total of five liters over the time of one minute—more than a gallon—against the resistance of the circulatory bed. Even at rest the heart delivers a total volume of blood that could fill up a fifty-five-gallon drum in less than an hour. The cardiac muscle fibers themselves are specialized, unique within the body. At the microscopic level, they share some structural features with skeletal muscle, but they are involuntary, like the smooth muscle in blood vessels, the stomach, the uterus, the iris, and hair follicles. Seen under an electron microscope, cardiac fibrils branch—another unique feature—but have tight junctions between them to keep them from ripping apart as they strenuously work.

In addition to the upper and lower way of dividing the heart conceptually, there's the side-by-side view. The right heart (with stacked atrium and ventricle) sends blood to the lungs; the parallel left heart must pump against higher pressure to the entire body; therefore, it has thicker walls. When a patient has end-stage left-heart failure, he or she may have a mechanical device implanted, an LVAD (Left Ventricular Assist Device) as a temporizing measure that can bridge the patient over until cardiac transplantation.

When cardiologists assess the heart sounds, they can hear in remarkable detail problems of the heart's action. A mechanical heart sound simulator is used at some medical schools; it is capable of reproducing some twenty-five abnormal sounds, thus giving doctors-in-training practice in hearing the signs of a "patient" who cannot die. Dr. Hardy, who has listened to thousands of hearts, believes that the sounds of Michael's heart suggest that the aortic valve is bicuspid, with two leaflets instead of the normal three. By this theory, the malformation is congenital; Michael's heart has worked for twenty-six years but is now wearing out, no longer stopping backflow or regurgitation; it's not healthy enough to serve his entire body. But only direct observation during the operation will give the truth of the valve's state.

The critical measurement here is the *ejection fraction,* the percentage of blood that is expelled from the left ventricle with each contraction, calculated by echocardiography, an ultrasonic exploration of the heart. The technician I observe sits at a boxy machine housing a computer and an ultrasound generator; she moves a transducer over a patient's chest as the patient lies on her side. The transducer looks like a microphone on a cord attached to the machine, but while a microphone only receives sound waves, the transducer sends out sound waves and then receives their echoes, like the sonar of a bat or a submarine. The computer converts these sound waves into pictures on a monitor. Through the magic of computers, the signals from the heart can be stopped at various points of filling or emptying the four chambers. The technician adjusts measuring devices for these two images and the computer calculates the ejection fraction: for example, 50–55 percent would be the lower limit of a normal reading. A reading of 20 percent indicates that the heart's efficiency is severely reduced and the reason would be sought. The way blood comes from the heart is explored by hemodynamics, now a sophisticated study of the physics of turbulent and laminar flow, wave forms, and other arcana of dynamic fluid mechanics.

While less dramatic, the return of blood through the veins is equally important and in some ways more complicated. The blood needs to be recirculated, the carbon dioxide exchanged, and wastes removed by the liver. Some animals have multiple hearts to move blood back toward the heart, but humans have only the blood-dispersing heart. Furthermore, some of the blood plasma—now called lymph—leaks out of the capillaries to bathe cells, and it has no secondary heart to send it back. The answer, both for lymph and for venous blood, is the pumping activity of all our muscles and especially muscles associated with breathing; blood and lymph move slowly but steadily through one-way valves and are reunited in large veins just before reaching the heart. In a sense, the entire body constitutes a pump for these two fluids.

The metaphor of a pump compares the living, organic heart to a mechanical, typically metallic, object. Industrial pumps—especially in Harvey's day—were force pumps that functioned by a single energy source (electricity, steam, or a human hand) to move liquid, for example, water in coal mines. Like most metaphors, the heart-as-a-pump both clarifies some aspects of the heart and ignores, hides, or confuses others. First, the heart as a pump would be more accurately seen as *two* parallel pumps with two circulations, one to the lungs and one to the body. (Indeed, we could even claim a third circulation to the coronary arteries and veins.) Next, while the vasculature is a relatively closed system, the allied lymphatic system is not.

Furthermore, as we saw in Dr. Duran's lab, the heart is not just a force pump, but (very likely) also a suction pump. The heart is not, of course, a mechanical pump with metallic walls but a varying organ that can change its rate and amount of blood expelled in each beat. These variations come from the complex interactions of the two nervous systems and the biochemical messages that act on heart muscle. Thus the energy sources and controls are more complex than a steam engine. Finally, mechanical pumps have no minds, no ideas, no emotions, no imaginations, all of which we keep in our cultural hearts.

CORPOREAL DYNAMICS: HUMANS, LOBSTERS, BEARS

When I first met Michael I felt the urge to mention some physical shortcoming I had, to share my own parallel vulnerability and mortality. I didn't want to touch on my deep, existential angst, so I told him that I had lately had some trouble with my back.

"Tight hamstrings?" he asked immediately.

I had to think a minute. Stress on the lower back, I had reasoned, involved the torso, the stabilizing muscles of the stomach, flexibility of the spine, and so on. I never thought about being "locked up" from below, from the legs. But Michael was an experienced athlete who would know about such things. Due to travel, the "good life," and a vacation mentality, I had stopped doing a series of stretches I regularly did at home. One is the yoga posture called The Plow: you lie on your back and bring your feet up over your torso, over your head, and rest your toes in your hands stretched up past your head. After Michael's suggestion, I got on the floor in my Missoula apartment and made some tests. Sure enough, the hamstrings were tight. My knees wouldn't open as far as they should; furthermore, I could feel the pull on my lower back. The big muscles in the back of the thigh had shortened. I resolved to have them stretched out before Michael returned for his surgery.

While Michael was back in California, I had another corporeal adventure. My hospital and the university cooperate in sponsoring a wellness center which provides fitness testing. In the increasingly distant past, I was in good shape, a long-distance runner. I used to run 5Ks (five-thousand-meter races), 10Ks, half marathons, even a couple of marathons and a triathlon. My resting pulse was in the 40s and, for a young forties hotshot, everything seemed possible. That was twenty years ago; now I was twenty-five pounds heavier. Although I usually jogged, I had done nothing for ten weeks, and with the back trouble, I felt like an old man, thick in the middle. I could feel my balance changing: trying to get out of chairs, for example, had become a more difficult maneuver. Part of me assumed I was still a long-distance racer, a whippet, lean and lithe . . . a strong and flexible man. My clothes and my mirror told me something else: I was fat. I had a spare tire around my waist, the kind of body fat that suggests cardiac risk. The topic of personal space and body habitus became concretely real to me. Being chronically sick could be a basis for personal definition, perhaps as it was for my grandmother, the timorous heart patient. So I signed up for fitness testing.

Joan Edlund, a personal trainer, met me in a small concrete block room at the Field House. She hooked me up to her computer for a stationary bike ride, a biceps pull, and a spine flexibility test. She had me do push-ups and sit-ups.

She took my blood pressure and my pulse. She did skin-fold tests to measure fat under the skin. The computer cranked and printed out its judgment: in sum, I was physically unfit. One test came out great: the sit-ups. Makes sense, I thought; this was the one thing I had been pretty faithful about. Other factors: I got nervous before such things, so pulse and blood pressure would be mildly elevated. Joan said, "Take your pulse when you wake up." I did; it was 64, not her 84. Body Mass Index calculations put me on the borderline of healthy, not her 25 percent fat, so I was suspicious of the accuracy of the skin-fold test. But—all quibbling aside—I knew I was some fifteen pounds overweight and somewhat out of shape. My legs were strong from years of racing and even jogging, but my arms, my flexibility, and now my aerobic capacity lagged behind.

Fortunately, St. Patrick Hospital provides a small gym free of charge to its employees. Joan met me there and showed me what exercises to do in what order. Several times she told me to slow down, as I revealed my Type A personality. She put me on various cardio machines, a treadmill, a climber, a rowing machine, and stationary bikes. In a couple of weeks I was stronger and down five pounds, my resting pulse was in the mid 50s, and my back stopped hurting. I felt a whole hell of a lot better. The human body was made for action; when it sits at desks all day, sits at computers, rides in cars, sits to watch television, puts the garbage down the sink instead of in the can outside, and so on, it gets stiff, out of shape, and the mind can become cranky. But the body is also made for rest and repair. The heart's very rhythm illustrates the stroke/relax principle, a cycle of effort and regeneration.

Occasionally, I see a golden eagle overhead or a bear roaming into town, and every evening, I spot deer in the mountains beyond Missoula. I think about the hearts of such creatures. What are they like? How do they work? How are they like the hearts of humans? I take a trip to the Mansfield Library on campus and learn that the development of hearts over biological time parallels the evolution of all living creatures. The simplest single-cell organisms floated in the ocean, which provided (straight through the cells' walls) gases and nutrients, as well as a sink for dispersal of wastes. As animals became more complex, with more cell layers and more distance to traverse, various systems evolved to move fluids along through the organism: sinuses, simple hearts, and two-, three-, and four-chambered hearts. Hearts for each species have developed to meet the needs for that species; or, in more Darwinian terms, only the hearts that worked for particular niches survived.

Biologists divide circulation in the animal world into two major kinds: open and closed. Closed is what humans have, with blood all contained in fine plumbing. An open system allows bloodlike hemolymph to bathe internal organs, with various sinuses and hearts to pump it along. This is a low-pressure, low-speed system, more an ooze than a flow. Flatworms have a single gastrovascular cavity for food and hemolymph combined. Clams and other bivalves also have an open system, with a heart beating at a very slow 10 to 20 bpm (beats per minute). Lobsters have an open system with a single-chambered but valved heart that runs at about 100 bpm, although the pulse is temperature dependent. (In the cooking pot, obviously, the temperature will exceed the heart's ability to survive.) Squids and octopi have closed systems with three hearts working away at a lower pressure than ours, just 60/40 mm/Hg (millimeters of mercury, compared to a typical 120/80 human range). Fish, as we know from cleaning them, have a low blood percentage, about 5 percent, as opposed to the 6 to 10 percent in birds and mammals. Fish have two-chambered hearts, and their gills are included in a "single circuit" (not a double circuit which includes a set of lungs). Most amphibians have three-chambered hearts and two circuits. Birds and all mammals (including humans) have four-chambered hearts and, of course, a double circuit. Indeed, one biology text says that all mammals' hearts are "essentially the same."

Pulse rates vary widely, especially with highly active creatures such as small mammals and birds. A squirrel monkey's pulse is reportedly between 360 and 410 beats per minute. A robin pumps away at some 570 bpm, and a blue-winged teal has been measured at 1,000 bpm. Perhaps the champion for the range of highs and lows are bats, who pump at 600 bpm when active (that's ten beats per second; try tapping your finger on the table that fast) but only 10 to 16 bpm when at rest, or roughly 2 percent of the active rate. Bears—even though famous for hibernation—lower their pulses to just 10 percent of active rate; some scientists call this torpid state drowsiness or "adaptive hypothermia" rather than true hibernation. By contrast, a ground squirrel lowers its rate from 150 to 5—a true hibernation. The world's smallest mammal, a shrew, has a heart the size of a grain of rice that zips along at 800 to 1,000 bpm.

Comparative studies show differences in the amount of blood moved, expressed in liters per hour. The slow-moving dogfish and shark average 7.5. A resting hen does about 24. A human pumps 280—equaling about 75 gallons, if it could be gathered as one amount. (This hourly rate is about 4.5 liters per minute; Dr. Oury estimated that Michael would be capable of 8 liters per minute at rest, or high normal.) A giraffe—with its large bulk and the elongated neck—must circulate some 1,200 liters per hour. Indeed, the giraffe has one of the toughest circulatory jobs, raising blood some ten feet up the neck to the brain. It has, therefore, a large heart, as large as an elephant's, some fifty pounds. It works at a very high blood pressure (260/180), with a specialized valve system in the neck to keep blood flow steady, whether the head is up to feed in trees or low to drink from a stream. A heart that big doesn't need many beats: 60 per minute will do. Elephants pump (at rest) just twenty-five times a minute.

Marine mammals, such as dolphins and whales, are especially interesting, because they have the lung development of land animals but later adaptations for the cold environment of the deep sea. Dolphins have an arterial sleeve over veins to heat blood returning from ocean-cooled flippers. (Some land animals also have circulation systems geared especially to heat dissipation; the Thompson's gazelle in East Africa has a loop of vasculature up into its horns to cool blood heated by, say, a hard run.) Seals can lower their blood pressure by 90 percent. Porpoises and manatees can selectively lower blood pressure in small arteries, while maintaining normal circulation to brains and lungs. Turtles, when diving, can do a cardiac shunt to cut off the lungs temporarily, yet Humboldt and emperor penguins (described as "hard to test" in the water) change their circulation very little during dives. Whales have an immensely large volume of cells needing blood, of course, and they dive to depths of several atmospheres of pressure. What kind of heart can manage these demands? In *Among Whales* (New York: Scribners, 1955) Roger Payne writes: "In a large blue whale the heart weighs about four thousand pounds (that's two tons) and probably pumps about sixty gallons with each beat. Its valves would be about the size of a hub cap, and a child could crawl through the aorta, the large blood vessel of the heart." Such a mighty heart, at maximal effort, would need to contract "only about 18 to 20 times a minute, or once every three seconds."

The *heartedness* of all creatures is amazing in its diversity, powerful in the similarities. If we could hear them all beating at once—encircling the globe, on land, in the air, in the rivers, lakes, and seas—a vast percussion of life, could we bear the sound? Even just by being more aware of them, can we learn some lessons that might extend, even save our lives? If so, wouldn't we be better able to protect the futures of all creatures? Or, if the human race disappears (because of a nuclear war, a vast plague, crop blights, pervasive biochemical pollution, an asteroid?), the rest of nature will just carry on without us, as it has for billions of years before the very strange experiment of the large-brained (but sometimes stupid) Homo sapiens, just now six billion strong, having doubled in my lifetime. But, bleak thoughts aside, our hearts and our bodies work—on the whole—very, very well. How did we develop the hearts we have?

Needing help, I call up my friend Dann Siems, an evolutionary biologist in Bemidji, Minnesota, whom I know through the Society for Values in Higher Education. I vaguely remember a phrase from a distant biology course, "ontogeny recapitulates phylogeny." Dann explains: Ernst Haeckel (a German biologist and philosopher who died in 1919) promoted the idea that the "higher" mammals represented, in their embryological development, all previous forms of life, from single-cell creatures, through fish and amphibians, right on "up." He presented a series of photos showing striking similarities between embryos of humans and the embryos of other animals. The motto he coined to summarize this notion was, indeed, "ontogeny recapitulates phylogeny," or "growth of an individual [human] sums up the development of all previous species." The idea was not only attractive but influential: humans were seen as the pinnacle of evolution, the summative being whose corporeal wisdom had outgrown and subsumed all earlier forms. Now, however, biologists see the concept applying only to the earliest events in embryo development, because various creatures branched off into their own species-specific structures that do not appear in human embryology. (Furthermore, it appears that Haeckel fudged in his selection of photographs, leaving out ones that didn't illustrate his contention.)

A paradox, then. My heart, Michael's heart, your heart, all human hearts beat in parallel fashion with all other hearts, be they insect, marine, reptilian, avian, or mammalian, and yet each species has developed variations appropriate to its own activities. Indeed, Dann says, the Haeckelian motto can provide insight when reversed to "phylogeny recapitulates ontogeny" (as Walter Garstang suggested as early as the 1920s), meaning that a species only exists retrospectively. Only after enough individual creatures have grown up as, say, striped bats or fulvous baboons can we call them a species. The driving force is the DNA shifts that create genetic variations, which the environment selects or suppresses, as Darwin saw it. Darwin, however, had a deistic notion of species as entities, ideal categories of potentials to be realized. Modern biologists, by contrast, see a gigantic gambling game of genes and habitats. For the heart, Dann tells me, the subtle variations in its structure—and therefore function—arose from variations in the processes of cell division and differentiation. And then the animal test drives the heart in nature to see whether it works, whether it will be passed on to offspring.

Are humans, then, just another set of gamblers amidst chemical pollutions, urban stresses, warfare, global warming, and yet-unknown factors? There are variations in hearts, some of which work fine for decades before failing, some of which end lives in the womb or on the basketball court. One evening my friend Charles died in his easy chair at age forty-two. The autopsy showed a heart malformation; the doctor said, "He was lucky to live that long." Do his children carry their mother's cardiac genes (presumably normal), or his, which may also kill them in midlife?

If turtles and hummingbirds and giraffes have custom-made hearts (so to speak), how have human hearts come to be constructed and—if we can figure backward—for what purpose? Anthropologists say we developed over millennia for such activities as hunting and gathering, ranging over a habitat, and making long migratory treks. Early humans also experienced periods of intense activity alternating with periods of relaxation. By some estimates they needed only about 25 percent of their waking hours to provide for their need for food. The rest of the time could be for play, social activities, grooming, telling stories, interpreting dreams, studying, and (enjoying) nature. The heart that worked fine for thousands of generations under those conditions was not designed for decades of repetitive stress from working sixty-hour weeks, sitting at desks, commuting two hours a day, eating fatty, salty, refined foods, drinking too much alcohol, and smoking. The 250 years of the Industrial Revolution are much too brief a time for our hearts to have evolved to match our urban lives—if such a thing were possible. And conditions in which we live will probably change even faster over the next 250 years.

Our cardiac equipment, millions of years in the making, is the best possible for us, and a place of daily miracles. Each human heart comes together in the womb with—almost always—wonderful precision. In the earliest days of an embryo, the neural tube and the heart tube develop as the planar embryo bends its edges together; specialized cells must match up from two sides. (If all goes well, it's the beginning of the heart; if not, the fetus may develop with anomalies—some compatible with life, some not—leading to spontaneous abortion.) Cardiac jelly slowly makes the tube, which completely fuses about the twenty-third day of fetal life. The heart—even in this primitive form—starts to pulsate on day twenty-two, when the embryo is less than an inch long. The linear tube migrates into an S shape, and aortic arches form, the ur-stages of arteries. The tube twists and turns, deepening its concavities, which will become the four chambers when septation divides them. This heart takes care of fetal circulation, bypassing the fetal lungs until birth, when the ductus arteriosus abruptly closes and the infant's lungs suddenly take over. Sometimes the ductus does not fully close (a condition called patent ductus arteriosus or PDA, one cause of "blue babies"), but surgery can now quickly fix this defect. Indeed, it is both common and remarkably successful, one of the cardiac surgeries with the best long-term results: little kids heal wondrously well. I've seen three-day-old premies go for this surgery and come back to their isolettes to continue their maturation without, it seems, missing a beat.

I also remember my daughter's birth vividly, even after almost thirty years, her blue-gray skin, her flaccid body as she came out. Dr. Southerland drew her high in the air, the umbilical cord dangling back to Nancy. He held the baby's ankles in one of his hands and flicked the soles of the feet with the fingernails of his other hand. She jerked, breathed, and cried the small, jerky bleat of infants. Her body stiffened and jumped, and her skin suddenly turned pink as her heart kicked into its new circulation pattern, one that lasts a lifetime.

Looking into the Heart

Michael's still back in California; from time to time he donates blood to be sent up for his operation. While I wait for his return, the word "stethoscope," with its root sense of "looking into the chest," is on my mind. When I observed in Radiology at the University of North Carolina, Chapel Hill, I was fascinated by how doctors could convert gray shadows into medical facts, imaginatively expanding two dimensions into three, listing the five possible causes (and their order of likelihood) of an abnormal finding, and suggesting the next one or two tests that would narrow the diagnosis. With a one-second look, a veteran radiologist can say, "This is a normal chest," dismissing scores of things that can go wrong with heart, lung, stomach, muscle, gut, liver, spleen, rib, vertebra, spinal cord, vasculature, and lymphatic ducts. The cardiac silhouette alone can show congenital deformities or, as in Michael's case, selective hypertrophy or abnormal growth to compensate for loss of function. Michael has mentioned the echosonography for his heart; how do medical professionals perceive the heart through technology?

Jim Thomas, R.T.N., agrees to show me around the Radiology Department at St. Patrick Hospital. Given that there's a long tradition in medicine that workers—whether technicians, technologists, nurses, or doctors—explain their craft to premed students, med students, and visiting professionals, he is glad to host a visitor interested in his work. This will be no leisurely tour, however. Today, as usual, the staff is at work diagnosing sick patients' hearts.

We enter a dimly lit room. Jim gestures to a chair in front of the largest computer monitor I've ever seen. On the screen are rows of circles about a half an inch wide, with a rainbow of colors in each circle. They have an eerie beauty all their own, quite apart from their utility: the circles on the screen are sections of heart walls, as if the heart has been cut across in slices.

"That's the guy over there," Jim says, pointing to an elderly man lying on a raised bed, his nose pointing toward the ceiling. Above him are two panels side by side and angled like the roof of a small house. Jim explains that these panels receive gamma rays emitted from radioactive chemicals in the man's heart, relaying this information to the computer, which creates the imagery on the monitor. Because these panels can move above the man, they can create various views of his heart.

"We want to see all walls pulling equally. That's the beauty of 3-D," Jim says. "This is SPECT, or Single Photon Emission Computed Tomography," he explains. "We stick the radioactive chemicals into the patient, let them circulate the right amount of time, then see what those panels overhead will pick up. The panels are gated, which means they're synchronized to collect information at the same, repeated point in the heart's cycle of activity—otherwise, we'd have a big blurry mess. This way we can pretend the heart is standing still, even though we know the patient is alive. The computer churns and clunks, and we get the array of 'slices' here. 'Tomography'—from the Greek *tome* for 'a cutting' and *graphein* for 'to write'—means 'cuts that are written.'" He chops the air with a flat hand. "You can print it all out, if you want, although it isn't as clear. The colors give gradients of saturation of the chemicals in our hearts. What we want to see is equal colors showing equal activity."

I'm still confused about the 3-D. Clearly the monitor's screen is 2-D.

Jim explains. "Sure, the screen if flat, but those panels can move to thirty positions, so we get different views of the heart. Watch this." He twiddles some controls, and the circles undulate in position on the screen.

Pointing to a shadowy part of one circle, I have the strange feeling I'm putting my finger in that man's heart. "What's this?" I ask.

"We call that 'a bite out of the doughnut.' It shows a defect in the heart. It means the panels aren't reading much at that point—the chemicals are only sparsely there, which means that blood isn't circulating well there. He has some kind of ischemic heart disease right there. We can describe it rather precisely. And then the docs will know what to do—to balloon an artery, or rotoblade it open, or stick in a stent—a metal tube that'll keep it open—or open him up and do a CABG." (CABG means coronary artery bypass graft; medical people usually pronounce it "cabbage.")

"And the parallel lines?" I point to the two similar series of slices on the monitor.

"One set shows our readings of the heart at rest, and the other shows the same areas under stress. Some people do fine with light activity, but feel pain going upstairs, say. We can find out why. That's the glory of nuclear medicine."

I'd seen stress tests . . . indeed, I'd taken one myself some years ago. When an EKG during a routine physical suggested the possibility of a mini block in my left anterior descending coronary artery, my doctor, Rick, said we should see whether it meant anything under stress. Wearing my shorts and running shoes, I was led into a small room dominated by a treadmill. Cold air rushed out of the ceiling. "Cold in here," I said. "You'll be glad in a moment," Rick said. A technician put the EKG cups on my chest and I got on the machine. I walked, then jogged, then ran. I heated up and was indeed glad for the Niagara of cold air pouring over me. Rick raised the front of the treadmill until I felt, sweating away, as though I were running straight up a mountain. He scanned the EKG strips, drawing the ribbons of paper through his hands while I toweled off and wondered whether my heart was OK. Rick concluded that it was fine. This was years ago, before I gained proficiency as a cardiac worrier, so this good news didn't have much impact on me at the time—I took it for granted. Now, I look back and derive some comfort—however outdated—from it. I look around for a similar treadmill and see none. "How do you stress people here?"

"I'll show you in a minute. It's really neat." While Jim turns to some of the tasks he must do today, I scan the room. A bulletin board displays some examples of office humor. "The beatings will continue until morale improves," reads one. Another states, "When I die, I want to do so peacefully like my grandfather, not screaming like the passengers riding in his car." And "Please be seated; the doctor is way behind schedule; sleeping bags and emergency rations are available from the receptionist." While patients are stressed in many ways, medical workers are stressed in others—perfectionism, perceived battles with death, legal liability, pecking orders between professions, rivalry between services, bureaucratic structures, and more. The bulletin board's contents are stress-relievers for Jim and his colleagues, and I admire how the doctors here apparently appreciate satire.

Another man in a white coat stops by and Jim introduces me to his boss, Dr. Allan Gabster. I say how impressive the sights on the monitor are.

"Imagery like this is much better than actually opening up a chest," Dr. Gabster says. "Nukes give us a lot more information. Diagnostics are so good now that there are few postmortems. If anyone dies of heart disease after this workup, we usually know why. We view a postmortem as a loss, anyway," he says with the bravura of a man used to saving people's hearts. "Our business here is *function*," he says with pride. "X-rays can give you structures, but we can show whether something is *working* or not."

Jim takes me to the corner of the room, where a smaller inset room comprises the hot lab. It has lead shielding around it, because this is where the radioactive materials are stored and prepared. "We use technetium, which is a daughter product of molybdenum," he says. He explains some nuclear physics I can't entirely follow, except that hot particles in the bloodstream are not trapped by the lungs but are just right for entrapment in the heart. "Avid" is a wonderful word that's used for the heart's eagerness to catch the isotopes; the cardiac muscles are avid for certain radioactive materials, and human beings are avid for meanings, especially about life and death.

"Let's go next door," Jim says, and we walk down the hall toward another room. On our left are the MRI scanners. Someone opens a door and I hear the *rat-a-tat-tat* of the electromagnet's moving wires that form a tunnel; within, a patient lies on the narrow moveable table. (Some places use a hula hoop to make sure the fit will work.) Patients need to lie still for some forty-five minutes, depending on how many slices are made. The images come out with startling clarity, but, like X-rays, their advantage is in structure rather than in function. We turn right to enter another room, where an elderly woman lies on a bed, attended by technicians and Dr. Gabster. She looks nervous; her eyes dart around the room. "This is the pharmacological stress I was mentioning," Jim whispers to me. "We'll put some dobutamine into her and zip up her heart."

Dr. Gabster explains the procedure to her. "We'll give you some drugs to speed up your heart then ask you to squeeze this handgrip hard and fast. Then we'll take you next door to see how your heart is responding." She nods. A technician injects a syringe-load into her IV line. In a minute, her face turns pinker. Although lying flat on her back in bed, she's sweating.

"Oh, my," she says. "I can really feel my heart pounding!"

"That's very good," Dr. Gabster replies. "Just what we need." The pulse rate he wants should be 220 minus her age times 90 percent; if she's seventy, that would give a target of 135, which she could never reach on a treadmill. When she reaches her target pulse rate, they'll take her next door for the nuclear scan, and her two rows of polychrome doughnuts will appear on the big monitor, displaying the inner workings of her heart.

Tasting Heart

Radiology allows us to see the heart in wonderful, minute detail, but this vision is indirect, a radio-chemical-computer insight that appears evanescently on the pixels of the monitor's screen. Must there always be some translation, some metaphor, so that we perceive the heart only at one remove? Can the heart be directly apprehended? One answer is palpation, or feeling the heartbeats with the hand on the front of the chest. I think of Barbra Streisand's character in the movie *What's Up, Doc?* offering such precordial information to the eager men at her banquet table. But even such a direct sensation would represent an indirect knowledge of cardiac activity. What senses can we bring to direct experience? I have *seen* live hearts beating, but only on television or videotape. I have also *seen* dead hearts in various anatomy labs. I have *touched* cadaveric hearts with my fingers, feeling their chambers and valves. I have *heard* my own heart beating through a stethoscope or in times of stress, but I can't sense it now, nestled between my lungs, protected by my sternum, ribs, and vertebrae, although I have every confidence that it resides there.

What about smell and taste? No one in the anatomy labs would *eat* an embalmed heart, although the unpleasant smell comes from the preservation, not the meat itself. I have *eaten* beef heart in the past at a Latin festival in the

Adams-Morgan section of D.C.; it's a favorite of Ecuadorians. But that was some years ago. What's available today? We read of tribes that seek the qualities of their vanquished enemies by eating their brains and hearts. Whose heart would I wish to eat?

The question becomes moot when Dixie McLaughlin, my administrative director at the Institute of Medical Humanities, offers me some pickled deer heart. Dixie's family has hunted each fall for years, butchering the take to fill their freezer. They consider pickled deer heart to be a delicacy. I think this may be in part a test of visiting Floridians . . . but I'm willing to try it.

The next day she brings in a Mason jar to work with many strange brown slices floating in clear liquid. I see allspice, bay leaves, and other spices I don't recognize. Does Dixie see doubt in my eyes? She suggests I try it on crackers as an hors d'oeuvre, and I take the bottle home to show my wife. "Not right now," she says. Although she was raised on a farm and has cleaned and cooked all sorts of wild game, this trophy evidently goes beyond some pale.

The following day Dixie asks me for my report. I admit the bottle wasn't opened.

The next night I know I must do better, so I crank off the lid and take out some slices, smelling a pleasant vinegary-spicy odor. The slices seem to have been made through the raw heart horizontally, like the latitudinal doughnuts of the SPECT. I find a small piece that appears to be the end, or the apex of a heart. It reminds me of the peaks of some local mountains. I fish out the largest piece and find the flattened holes of the chambers; these shapes make sense: in death, the heart would not expand in order to pump. The smooth curves certainly do not suggest a metallic pump. The meat itself is fine-grained, dark brown, with no fat anywhere. (Almost all wild game, except bear, is low in fat: fat animals can neither catch other animals nor escape predators.) I nibble a piece and find it delicious, tangy and just a bit chewy. My wife consumes a token bit.

The next day I tell Dixie—before she can quiz me—of my enjoyment.

"It's not for everyone," she replies, "but we really like it." She goes on to describe how they hang a dead deer in their garage, with the door well locked. Some neighbors in Missoula have lost game or hides to animals, possibly mountain lions. In several evenings, often with beer or sherry, I consume all the rest of the pieces. Will this make me deerlike? Give me antlers? More soberly, I think about this heart powering a deer—like the mule deer and white tails that appear on Mt. Sentinel behind us every evening—helping it run over hill and dale, jumping effortlessly over fallen trees or fences. I think about the events that ended this deer's life, and how Dixie's family, her neighbors—indeed all hunters, human or animal—are seekers of hearts.

Dixie has been telling me about a yearly event at the university, a dinner of wild game. My wife and I invite another couple and show up at a ballroom in the student union.

Upon entering, we find a large deer hanging from the ceiling on a long chain. Since the chain goes around the eight-pointed antlers, the rest of the deer hangs down, head to tail, suggesting one etymology for "barbeque": "barbe à queue" ("beard to tail"). A neat plastic tarp below him catches dollops of blood. This stag is mostly skinned and partly butchered, with large slabs of red meat hanging off it. A bandana tied around the stag's neck (to cover the gunshot wound, I later learn) does not have the same endearing effect as on pet dogs or the stylized images of howling coyotes we see in gift shops. Indeed, the entire picture is profoundly unappetizing. Nonetheless, we press on and take our seats in the rows of chairs facing a stage.

The first speaker is a hunting enthusiast. It seems to me that no one has told him that this is a crowd in Montana (where almost everyone hunts and fishes) or a university crowd (which prefers a modicum of sense); he goes on a rambling tirade against "hunter haters" who wish to "ban hunting, take away our guns," and "take away our rights to fresh game, which has the distinct taste to be found nowhere else." The next three speakers put on demonstrations of food preparation, using an overhead video camera and a huge screen. The two men and one woman are deft, clear, and often funny as they prepare their dishes. Contrary to the first speaker's claim, these recipes are complex, apparently designed to disguise the flavor of gamy meats. Nor is economy of time a virtue . . . the three hundred of us waiting know that there are four buffet lines behind the screens to our immediate left. Through a set of room dividers we catch glimpses of various helpers carrying out large, mysterious dishes. My stomach growls.

After a discussion of the various exhibits that line the room for visiting after dinner, the crowd is finally released to eat. We surge forward, calculating which line will sate us the most quickly. When I reach the tables, I am delighted at the offerings and pile my plate high. There are Elk Meatballs over Wild Rice, Marinated Bear Noisettes, Mountain Lion Pierogies, John's Coffee Duck, Bear Geschnitzeltes and Spaetzle, and another half a dozen dishes. I take samples of each and return to my place. Almost immediately, I'm full. I'm ashamed that I have taken too much, allowing my eyes to want everything, my hunger to demand a lot, my penchant for research to overcome my habit of eating little meat, and my ignorance of the nature of game meats. Wild game provides a dense meat, solid protein with very little fat. The venison meatballs in particular are dry and very filling; I learn later that some cooks mix deer meat with beef, pork, or lamb—anything with some fat content. The only meat I really like is the bear meat, which is the greasiest, that is, more like the meats Americans usually eat. Bears need to "feed up for the winter," as some locals say, storing huge amounts of calories as fat throughout their bodies. Dixie later tells me that some people (including her) won't touch bear meat, knowing that bears are omnivores, eating virtually anything, including small game, roots, wild honey, and huge amounts of huckleberries. Indeed, bears have been troublesome this year, owing to a thin huckleberry crop in the uplands and increased harvesting by humans to make pies and jams. So bears have ranged further down into the valleys, raiding dumpsters and any human food left unguarded. Bears love human food, which is almost always richer in fat than anything they can find in nature. Rangers tell us "A fed bear is a dead bear," meaning that bears fed by humans, accidentally or on purpose, will seek human food in the future, cause trouble, and have to be destroyed. Some are transferred to other territories, but their bad habits go with them, and they typically get into trouble (by human definition) again. Bears have destroyed all sorts of food containers—cans, picnic chests, even car doors and trunk lids—to get at food. They have broken into cabins. They have turned over outhouses and eaten the human waste beneath. Upon learning this, I join Dixie in her resolve.

But taboos are selective, socially learned, and arbitrary in many ways. What's vile to society is business as usual in the woods, where nutrients of all sorts are routinely recycled by animals, birds, fish, maggots, bacteria, and everything else. It's only humans who are preposterously wasteful; it's humans who have forgotten that their very name, "human," is related to the word "humus," or soil. In many places, Montana included, the loss of habitat and the stress of surrounding humans make life less possible for birds, fish, mammals. And, to the extent that we cannot live with other creatures, our own lives are (or will be) endangered.

What is the nature of the heart? It's part of the nature that surrounds me here in the Rockies, the nature that surrounds all of us, wherever we live, and the nature of our fellow creatures, all sharing the basic elements that make up nature—hydrogen, oxygen, nitrogen, and carbon—from rocks to rodents, clouds to crows, hills to humans.

VALVE JOB AT THE VALVE SHOP

Michael Flies In . . . Also His Parents (Tuesday, October 27)

It's freezing this morning, and my wife Nancy and I look out the back window and see the fog rolling down from Mt. Sentinel. The weatherman says that cool air descends from the mountains and pools in the valley "like a brick." While we read the paper over breakfast, the fog covers the golf course behind us, right up to our windows. Life in these mountains is different every day.

I'm excited: today's the day Michael arrives. In my Type-A vision of things, he'll fly in, have all his briefings, and go to the OR for surgery. He'll tell me all about it at supper time. I'll write it up this evening, and we'll discuss it over breakfast the next day.

I drive to the hospital with various thoughts swirling in my head. *I want to see Michael, simply because I enjoy his company. I don't want to see Michael because I don't want to be a parasite, a scavenger, a voyeur. I want to see Michael because he is articulate and witty. I don't want to see him because I might be a jinx on this whole project: Howard wants to write it up; therefore, Michael spits out blood in the OR, covering everybody and everything. He dies and comes back to haunt Howard's computer, word-wrangling faculty, and soul.*

I call up Carole to ask about his schedule and when I can say hello.

"Well, it looks like the fog is lifting, so I think they'll be able to land OK," she says. She coordinates patient visits from all over the world and knows what obstacles there can be. Late fall can be tricky, with fog, rain, and snow, although winter, of course, is the most difficult season. Michael's parents are coming in about noon, Michael later in the afternoon. He'll have a cardiac cath tomorrow and various bits of patient education. The surgery, with Dr. Duran and Dr. Oury, will occur Thursday morning. Michael will be intubated at least until that evening and sent to surgical intensive care for recovery.

Preparations for Surgery (Wednesday, October 28)

I go to the hospital early and head up to the Heart Institute on the fourth floor. I speak with Kim, one of the schedulers, and sit down in the lobby at a card table where the same jigsaw puzzle lies out. Some busy hands have been here in the last three weeks, leaving, of course, the toughest parts. Never mind. *Compulsives do good work,* I always say. I study the garish picture of leaping whales, a tropical island, and, below water, sea creatures of every hue. I start to study the still disconnected pieces. Each time the elevator door opens I look over expectantly. Each time, no luck. Back to the puzzle; no one has seen connections between two clusters of pieces assembled outside the frame and the remaining internal gaps. I transport the clusters inside (my sister liked to use a pancake turner) and triumphantly link them up. Is closing a surgical wound anything like this?

Before long Michael and his parents step out of the elevator. Michael seems taller than before and, upon seeing me, immediately opens his briefcase and pulls out a clipping. It's about Arnold Schwarzenegger, who has had the Ross surgery, a fellow athlete and now a model, even a guardian spirit. I meet Michael's parents, Kevin and Jayne. We converse about Montana and Minnesota. I remember the elevated "tunnels" between buildings in Minneapolis and ask about them.

"Oh yes, the skyways," Kevin says. "Very useful in the winter. You can go to a million stores and never go outside."

"Did you ever keep gerbils . . . as a kid?" Michael asks. I didn't, but I recall the cages with tubes for the little furry guys. "All that's missing is the wheel."

We all laugh.

I explain about my project and say how grateful I am to get to know Michael, avoiding the obvious medical phrase "to follow his case." Michael invites me to observe "anything going on today," and I thank him but decline. I still think my role is to wait until everything has gone well.

Katie Mackey, R.N., joins us. She has spent hours on the telephone with the Curry family. Kevin doesn't connect the face and voice until he reads her name on her white lab coat.

"Oh, you're Katie Mackey! You were so helpful on the phone!" he says. He shakes her hand once again.

Michael's parents seem remarkably calm to me, given that their son will have his chest sawn open tomorrow, his heart stopped, and dramatic surgery performed upon his heart. Was the human body designed to undergo such manipulation? Perhaps not, but medicine has learned how to do such things anyway, cooperating with the capacities of the body to heal itself after such an invasion, such—in the medical term—an *insult*. What a paradox: mutilating to repair, wounding to heal.

Cardiac Surgery (Thursday, October 29)

The weather report says that Indian summer (a.k.a. bluebird weather) is definitely over and that winter-like weather has taken hold of western Montana. I look out and see that snow has fallen during the night down to about 3,500 feet, almost the level of the valley floor. When I go in to the hospital, my co-workers Kathy and Carol speak of actual snowflakes in the air when they left for the hospital about 7:00 A.M. The newspaper says that today is also the day John Glenn will be shot into space once again, part of a day-long media party of remarkable dullness. At 8:00 A.M. I'm just having breakfast and imagining that right about now a scalpel is making a seven-inch midline incision on the chest of a well-sedated Michael Kevin Curry. Before long the Sarns saw will vibrate through his sternum. I tap my own breastbone, finding it quite intact.

About 9:30 A.M. I head up to the surgical waiting room. The Currys, who arrived at 6:00 A.M. with Michael, are not there.

I head back to the office and review my notes from watching the videotape of a Ross surgery. I imagine the scene. Michael is intubated and anesthetized, lying on his back. Dr. Oury, wearing a headlamp to illuminate the operating field, cuts a straight line down the chest for the median sternotomy: he splits the breastbone vertically, sawing it from top to bottom. A steel retractor goes in this opening; when cranked, it pulls the two halves apart, giving a roughly five-inch square window. Under the bright lights, the moist red tissues contrast nicely with the dull green towels folded on the four sides. When the pericardium is cut open, the naked heart's action is dramatically visible. (In the video I saw, it filled most of the screen, larger than life.) After preparations for tubes to run from the heart to the heart-lung machine, a cold chemical solution—called *cardioplegia*—stops the action of the heart. This period of time is called "cross-clamp time," referring to the clamps that remove the heart from the normal blood flow. For this operation, that time will be about three hours, during which the heart-lung machine will take care of the necessary gaseous changes in the blood. Past societies assumed no heartbeat equaled death; for them, Michael would be dead. For us, he's dependent on life-support machines . . . medically suspended in a drug-induced hibernation. From all this he will have to be *weaned,* as if from a mother's breast.

Dr. Oury will cut the aorta just above the valve that has been failing, and he and Dr. Duran will peer in to inspect and weigh their options. If it's a valve repair, Dr. Duran will take the lead. If it's the Ross, it'll be Dr. Oury. Echo studies have previously given an idea of the relative sizes of the aortic valve and the pulmonary valve, so they know the match is good for the Ross. The heart muscle—relatively bloodless now—looks like uncooked chicken flesh. Proceeding with the Ross, they remove two valves, discard the faulty aortic valve, and prepare its root (where it came from) for the pulmonary valve to be moved over. It will be trimmed then fitted into place for sewing. The silver needle holders (which resemble needle-nosed pliers) hook the curved needle through tissues, then grasp it on the other side and pull it through. Surgeons can sew wonderfully, gracefully, deftly. (Our word *surgery* comes from Greek roots *cheiros* and *ergein,* meaning *hand work,* even *handiwork.*) The former pulmonary valve is lined up over the now bare aortic root suspended on some forty sutures surrounding it; it waits a few inches above its destination. When all is ready, Dr. Oury pushes it down the suture lines to its new home in the aortic position and ties it in, knot by knot. The valve is tested for tightness. Then the sterilized pulmonary valve (a homograft—from a deceased human) is sewn into the pulmonary position. Blood is progressively let back into the heart to test all the work for leaks. Warm cardioplegia (literally an oxymoronic phrase, because "cardioplegia" means paralyzing the heart) urges the heart to start beating again. The patient gets thirty minutes of rewarming, still on bypass. The aortic cross-clamp is removed. The surgeon inspects for any bleeders. The clamps are removed, and the cardiovascular integrity and action is restored. An echo reading shows how well the heart is performing. Another 120 or so sutures will help close all layers. Seven shiny wires will tie the breastbone back together; these show up well on X-rays any time later as white loops with the ends twisted, much like twist ties from a kitchen drawer.

My imagining over, I return to the surgical waiting room at 10:30 A.M. and find the Currys. Carole has been giving them a tour of the Heart Institute and even the medical library. I sit down and we make small talk about the operation, Montana, travel by car, the weather. There's a wonderful view of the valley from this fourth-floor perch; I can see snow on Mt. Lolo to the south. Kevin refers to the on-going operation as a valve job, proclaiming, "We looked around and picked the best valve shop." I know it's a joke of sorts, but I wonder to what extent he's hiding his worries behind it: an automotive shop is a known thing, and an engine is metallic, relatively indestructible.

The Children's Theater Workshop in town is presenting *Fiddler on the Roof*. Kevin wants to line up tickets. Jayne wants to wait until everything is settled with Michael.

"They're doing the Ross." Kip, a surgical nurse, has come out of the double doors to give us an update. Inspection made; decision taken. "Even a valve replacement might need revision in another twenty years," approves Kevin. Jayne says she thought it was going to be the Ross all along. The Ross will take longer, perhaps a total of seven hours. The Currys go to their lunch; I go back to my office.

1:00 P.M. We're up in the waiting room once again, this time with Carole Erickson. Kip comes out again: "They're warming up the heart." Jayne, a nurse, knows what that means and claps her hands.

Carole explains: "The work on the valves is done. He's going off bypass and they'll be closing. We might as well head downstairs, where we'll meet him."

I leave for my class at the university, promising to see them tomorrow in the Special Care Unit, where Michael will be recovering.

Special Care (Friday, October 30)

It is truly fall today, with leaves flowing out of trees onto lawns, cars, the street. It is eighteen degrees when I look out this morning. A dog or coyote chases deer on the frosty slopes of the mountain behind us, with no success. I follow him with binoculars, so interested as to stand on my back stoop barefoot, in my pajamas. The dog-like thing is running hard, but the deer scatter before him effortlessly. They curl around to stop and stare back at him as he picks still others to chase. The mountain that has been picturesque—a place for us to view sunsets and turning leaves—is also a location for blood sports. I half wish to see the dog-thing make a kill, half wish to see the deer escape amidst raucous deer laughter. (Later, I learn from a wildlife biologist that it was probably a dog; so inefficient or even stupid was its behavior; he called it a "subsidized predator," with an easy meal waiting at home.)

Blood. I don't think about it much, but I carry some thirteen or fourteen pints, and my heart circulates it to the cells in my body. Michael has sent up three or four pints for his surgery. I wonder how much bleeding he did today. The videotape of the Ross procedure shows the suction wand entering the picture many times.

I scrape the heavy frost off the car's windows and drive in.

A hospital volunteer at the desk checks the roster for Special Care, looks at my name badge, and pokes a round plate on the wall. The automatic doors open inward, an aortic valve to my bloodlike entrance. The inner wall of Michael's room is clear glass, so nurses can see in easily. The outer wall has a window looking out into brilliant gold leaves, some sifting down through the others.

And there's Michael, flat on his back, his eyes closed. He has a tube in his mouth (his ventilator) and one in his nose (to decompress his stomach). He looks rather pale, somewhat gray, but mostly asleep. He said to his parents that he'd have the easiest time of all of us, because he'd be unconscious. I hope that's true. They're off making a phone call, the nurse tells me. I depart.

"Michael, can you hear me?" It's Dr. Oury by the bed at 2:30 in the afternoon. "Michael, wake up. As soon as you wake up, we'll have that tube out of your nose."

A nurse is at the foot of the bed. I'm outside the room. "And tomorrow," Dr. Oury continues, "we'll have you walking."

Dr. Oury comes out of the room and greets me. "He's doing great. The operation went perfectly for six hours, just what you like to see. We had a small bleeder this morning and we had to clean that up. It's hard on the family, though, after the big emotions. They often expect the worst when we have to go back, but it's usually very fast. We find the bleeder right away, patch it up, and we're done."

So . . . Michael had to go back in for a second operation. I bet that scared his folks, all right.

I knock. Jayne, on a stool at the bedside, smiles. I think of the many times she sat by his bed when he was a child. A nurse is at the end of the bed, stimulating Michael's toes.

"How're you doing?"

"Fine, we're doing fine!" Jayne says with a smile. She seems much relieved. Michael still looks pale to me.

"Michael, Howard's here. You should get those tubes out of you so he can interview you!" She grins broadly.

We laugh.

Michael raises his left hand in the air and slowly waves it back and forth. The sight gives me much joy.

"I'll be by tomorrow," I say.

Saturday, October 31, Halloween

Intensive Care Units constitute an eerie world of separation, isolation, and intensification of medical technology. The patients are typically passive, due to illness and/or sedating drugs; they have a profusion of tubes, lines, and sensors attached to them. In most ICUs the lights are on twenty-four hours a day, the doors always open. Patients can hear conversations and the beeps and honks of monitors. Sleeping is not easy. ICU psychosis, including hallucinations, is even possible; Christopher Reeve discussed his experience with this in his gripping memoir *Still Me* (New York: Random House, 1998). Visitors who have never seen such a place often find it overwhelming, frightening. As we are all mortal, patients and visitors up here are of many sorts: I see overalls, cowboy hats, and baseball caps with a variety of slogans for athletic teams, local industry, even a bar in Miles City, Montana, about six hundred miles away. I see weather-beaten faces, faces near tears, faces showing relief that the worst is over. The pay phone is often busy. People speak into it earnestly, sometimes gesturing with their hands, sometimes with notes before them to get everything right. Some of them are crying. Others are joyful.

For patients, it's a never-never land, an enforced hibernation. Many remember little about it. Others, as they emerge from sleep, ask profound questions about their lives. Some make an "ICU promise" (as one man put it) to fulfill when (or *if*) they leave the unit alive. My friend Jill, who was in a terrible car wreck years ago, told me about "making deals with God in the back of an ambulance," including her choice to enter the nursing profession.

Others go to "the floor" for palliative care until their inevitable deaths. Still others die in the ICU, leaving only as corpses. When I visited my friend Don in an ICU, pervasive cancers were eating him up. His hair was gone from chemo, he'd lost a lot of weight, and his papery skin was white, not the Florida tan I was used to. "I'm bleeding internally," he said in a whisper. "They can't find where it is." I offered some words of understanding, words I felt were not adequate. "It's OK, though," he said. "I'm ready. Enough of this." He made a small gesture of his hand to indicate his high-tech surroundings. "I'm ready." And the next day he was dead. We don't talk much about willed deaths in this culture, since they appear to be betrayals of our mythos that everyone should live forever and in perfect health, but many older people stop eating and drinking when they're ready to die. In some cases, we might say, death is the cure for the illness. Some people die shortly after a spouse's death. In some cultures, a perfectly healthy person can take to a bed and die in twenty-four hours, if he feels he's been hexed. The surrender of the mind to death can, it seems, bring the body along quickly. Or is it only surrender? Acceptance? Celebration? Departure to adventure?

Michael is propped up a bit today. His nurse Tony is working on a spaghetti of lines around the top of the bed. The sun shines through the window; all the leaves have blown out of the tree.

"Hey man, how you doing?"

"I had a long night," Michael says slowly. He has a tube in his nose, but the vent tube is gone from his mouth.

"I'll bet you did. What can I touch?" I say, extending my hand. Michael raises his right hand with a red light aglow on his middle finger, a sensor for oxygen saturation in his blood. I think of E.T. We shake hands. He's one tired puppy; I know I shouldn't stay long.

"I hear you're getting up to walk today."

"Really?"

"That's what Dr. Oury said yesterday; you were just coming out of it." I worry that I shouldn't be discussing this. "Is that right, Tony?"

"Yep, that's what we're getting ready to do right now."

"Well, this guy's a track star. You'll probably have to hold him back."

I say goodbye and leave. It's a day of brilliant sunshine. My wife and I are going hiking.

For Halloween that evening, a group of four of us put on silly costumes and hand out candy to children, most of whom have no idea about the sainted dead we are nominally celebrating. I'm glad Michael isn't one of them.

On to the Floor (Sunday, November 1)

I stop at the lobby information desk to find out whether Michael is out of Special Care. I surely hope so, but the attendant says, "Still in 342." I take the stairs up there and walk to 342. It's empty. And dark. For a moment I have the strange feeling that Michael is not only gone, but dead; reason prevails and I ask a nurse.

"He's up in 459."

Hooray, I think. Going to the floor is an obvious step toward becoming well. Michael now has a real room with opaque walls and a door that can close, I think, as I take the stairs to his new floor.

I knock and wait for a response.

"Come in."

Michael has a regular bed, regular windows, several bouquets of flowers, and a fine jack-o-lantern with an asymmetrical smile.

"How you feeling?"

"More like a real person."

I ask about the pumpkin.

"That's my dad's way of coping. He likes to make things." I picture Kevin in his motel room butchering, scraping, carving. I wonder what the maid thought of all the fresh pumpkin detritus.

We chat about the smoke in the valley outside his window, how it was worse a decade ago and so on.

Michael says, "You know, I had my fifth-year college reunion before coming up here. It made some of my fellow alums nervous to think about heart surgery, mortality, and all that. Twenty-seven-year-olds don't give that sort of thing much thought."

Or people twenty years older, I think. By their fifties, though . . . the baby boomers will have a lot to think about besides their retirement programs.

I ask if he needs some reading materials. "I made it through a bunch of the *New York Times*, but it's still hard to hold up a book." We agree that, in a day or two, I'll bring *Into Thin Air*, Jon Krakauer's gripping account of a disaster on Mt. Everest.

We decide it's always good to read about people in more trouble than we are.

Shower! (Monday, November 1)

I knock at 459 and receive no answer. Through the crack I see the bed is empty; I hear water running. A nurse with a big smile comes up the hall to say that Michael is showering.

I come back in fifteen minutes. Jayne is helping Michael on with his TEDS, compression stockings; these help the return of venous blood to the heart when there's very little muscle activity, which ordinarily helps the low-pressure blood and lymph return up to the heart. With these stockings there's less risk for deep vein thromboses (DVTs), dangerous clots in the leg. While waiting in the hall, I take a close look at the bright red crash cart parked there. It looks like the wheeled tool chests mechanics use in garages, wonderfully practical, with six locked drawers of meds, tubes, and other supplies. On top is a defibrillator/pacer device, with cords ending in the paddles that will be applied to a patient's chest. There's paperwork—all ready to go—an elevator key, even a stopwatch. If my heart stops anywhere, I hope it's near one of these.

Soon Michael is back in bed.

"Wow, you got a shower?"

"I can't tell you how good that felt," he says with a big smile.

I hand him some books, which he holds over his belly while we talk.

"And a special heart?" I gesture to the red cloth heart sewn on the front of his hospital gown.

"Yeah, special status. All the heart patients get them. Something for your book."

"I'll put it in."

"It's only us, though. I haven't seen any lungs or spleens or stomachs or guts. Just us."

Michael is looking pinker today, but with his hemoglobin at just 8 (normal would be 12 to 17), he'll be transfused later today. He makes a small gesture with the books; Jayne reaches to take them from him. Evidently he's still too sore and/or weak to lift them to the windowsill nearby.

"They're going to make me walk pretty soon," Michael says. As if on cue, there's a knock at the door and a woman appears, pushing before her the largest walker I've ever seen, a series of metal bars that constitute a three-sided cage. There's a green cylinder suspended on the front, an oxygen tank.

"Hi, I'm Marge. Cardiac rehab!" she says with a big smile. The people I've met who work in rehab are always upbeat, infinitely energetic and encouraging. I imagine that she and Michael's track coach have some traits in common. I take my leave, glad that Michael is about to hit the road again, if not yet the carousel. The structures of his heart repaired, now it's time to urge it to regain dynamic function.

Why Is the Pumpkin Laughing? Heartfelt Words of Emotion

Dr. Oury speaks of the "big emotions" families feel during surgery. I've felt them myself, sitting in the surgical waiting room during a friend's surgery and during my wife's surgery. Feeling helpless, we imagine the best outcomes as well as the worst. Giving someone over to dramatic events—such as having his chest cut open and the heart stopped—gives one pause. Dr. Oury and his colleagues know this well and take steps to comfort the feelings of family. Doctors have learned to control their own emotions, in part because they have done procedures many times. For the family, however, it's often the first time, and much of it feels surreal. Kevin makes jokes about the valve shop. Jayne has been calm and gracious, controlled before and during the operation. After the surgery, however, she becomes jocular, telling Michael to wake up for an interview.

As an outsider, I'm unlikely to hear about Jayne and Kevin's deeper emotions, including the worries all parents would have for a son needing and getting medical help. Besides, we tend to keep emotions within, not mentioning them. Sometimes we feel emotions viscerally, in our guts and in our chests. We breathe faster. Our blood pressure rises; our hearts speed up. Appropriately, there are many expressions in our language touching on emotions and the heart.

Wear your heart on your sleeve, heartthrob, lose your heart to someone, tug or pull at the heartstrings, the way to a man's heart is through his stomach, steal someone's heart, melt my heart, heart-stricken, heartsease (peace of mind; also a wild pansy once thought to cure the discomforts of love), *ease your heart, heart-free* (i.e., not in love), *heartache, heartbreak, heartsore, heartsick, sick to the heart, heartrending, heart-stopping, heartfelt, heartwarming, after one's own heart, do one's heart good, with a song in my heart, change of heart, eat one's heart out, from the bottom of my heart, dear to my heart, close to my heart, an affair of the heart, crime of the heart, set your heart at rest, set your heart on something, to your heart's content, heart-to-heart talk, two hearts beat as one, heartless, cold heart, hardhearted.*

This group is approximate, even messy, just like the emotions of love and hate represented; it is also large, suggesting the prevalence of desire in our inner lives. Some of these touch on erotic desire; the phrase (*two hearts beat as one*) retains a sense of ideal courtly love. (One reason given for the custom of wearing the wedding ring on the third finger of the left hand is that the vein of love—*vena amoris*—was said to run directly from there to the heart.) But other phrases (*crime of the heart*) suggest wild, passionate love, even for dangerous people, or out-of-control obsession as in adolescent crushes (*melt my heart, heartthrob*). With strong emotions, there is risk. *Losing one's heart* suggests the threatening loss of rational control. We can be *heartbroken, heartsore, or heartsick*—especially if there is a betrayal of love. This is also the realm of valentines, the stylized heart transfixed by Cupid's arrow, an arrow of pleasure and/or pain. Candy "conversation hearts" are a more domesticated version, with mottoes printed on them.

The arts routinely deal with emotions. Ludwig von Beethoven wrote "Von Herzen zu Herzen" ("from heart to heart," meaning from his heart to ours) on the score of his massive *Missa Solemnis.* French-American artist Dominique Mazeaud calls herself a "heartist." In an article in *American Artist,* Timothy S. Solliday, a California painter, says that art should help "clean up the heart condition of mankind." American education, however, often cuts courses in the arts, dismissing them as frills.

Still other expressions (*coldhearted, heartless, hardhearted*) suggest an inhumane humanity. To be human is to have emotions.

"That's my dad's way of coping with emotions," says Michael, referring to the carved pumpkin in his recovery room. Kevin uses a knife to improve a somewhat spherical, somewhat hollow organic object, an analogue to the somewhat spherical, sometimes hollow organic object of his son's heart that someone else had cut into. As he works the pumpkin's face, Kevin's interpretation (or hopeful prophecy) is a smile.

WALKING QUIETLY

Tuesday turns out to be the last day of Indian summer in the northern Rockies. Because it is Voting Day, there are no classes at the university, and friends take my wife Nancy and me over Lolo Pass and into the wilds of Idaho. I'm not kidding about the wilds: the Selway-Bitterroot Wilderness is forested mountain, sparsely populated. Except for the highway, and some ugly clear-cuts, much is unchanged from when Lewis and Clark made their trips through here almost two hundred years ago. On an earlier trip we saw a black bear ambling along the road. Lolo Pass is about 6,500 feet above sea level, cool enough for patches of snow, especially in shady areas. (Paradoxically, there are also hot springs here, where Lewis and Clark and company bathed with much pleasure.) Higher up—on Lolo Peak (9,000 feet)—much more snow is starting to build up, creating the famous "base" that skiers look forward to. Stellar's jays fly away from the road, where they pick up grain fallen from trucks; their bright blue-purple feathers flash in the sun. Beyond the pass, the vegetation changes abruptly: it's more lush, more verdant here on the side fed by Pacific moisture. As we slowly descend down merging valleys, we join the Lochsa River, where it's sunny and warm. We hike up a tributary to some hot springs, where we bathe beneath blue skies and loll away the midday. Although I greatly enjoy the beauty, the mood, and the company, my thoughts keep turning back to Michael. He called yesterday to say he was getting turned loose from the hospital early; could we meet Friday afternoon?

Mammoth Drinks; No Moguls (Friday, November 6)

As I drive to Michael's motel on the banks of the Clark Fork, I try to think of the perfect place to go. Suddenly it's now like winter, gray and cold, with a formidable wind, rushing out of the Hellgate, a canyon to our east. Michael meets me in the lobby with a big smile. He's wearing a black leather jacket: evidently we're not staying here. I ask where he'd like to go, and he says the university.

Before long we're sitting in the student union. Michael looks up at Mt. Sentinel through a huge, south-facing window. The enormous room—often full at lunch—is now almost empty, with only six or eight students scattered through it. We're slurping from two enormous Jumba Juices, a commodity I've never heard of but something Michael was thrilled to find here. "We have them all over California," he says, treating me to about a quart of Passionate Pleasures.

We've barely sat down, and Michael is saying, "Walking quietly—I think that's the motto for the last few days. I went from all kinds of tubes and sensors in me, from having my eyelids taped down, to walking—all in twenty-four hours. The physical therapist—the one you saw—told me, 'don't work too hard; we'll just do some walking quietly.' I liked that phrase. So much of life is hectic."

"You had that walker contraption?"

"Yeah, but I tried not to use it—pride being a factor. But I had to. My balance wasn't good. We did three slow loops around the hall. It was pretty dull, except that I wasn't wearing any underwear. There was a guy going the opposite way around our loop. He had on one of those hearts on his hospital gown just like me. I felt he was like a brother—a fellow heart wanderer. Or wandering heart. You don't see anybody wearing a cloth pancreas. But the heart there's a reverence for it. Anyway, passing this guy on each lap stirred my competitive juices, and I tried to gain ground on him each time we met. I nicknamed him the self-pusher."

"What?"

"He pushed his IV pole himself. My Mom was pushing mine. That was something else he gave me to shoot for. I could still be a self-pusher and walk quietly, I figured. I was still having blood put in me, two more units, and packed red blood cells."

"You look right in the pink now."

"Yeah, thanks. I figured I had seven or eight tubes in me, a catheter, and a wire to my heart, which they pulled out the last day of the hospital—boy, did that feel weird, like my intestines being pulled out."

We suck on the straws extending from our mammoth drinks. I wonder how I'll eat any supper.

"The nurses checked on my breathing exercises for a while, then stopped when they saw I was faithful about them."

"What were they?"

"You have to suck on a breathing tube. You pull against resistance to re-expand your lungs."

"What are they telling you to do next?"

"I'm supposed to walk a lot, every day, a mile, adding on blocks. I can jog in a month. I have to get an echo in two or three months to clear me to run again. I'll do the echo back here again because I like these people. Besides, I want to go skiing in February; I have a buddy lined up to come. I can do cross country and gentle downhill. But no moguls."

"What?"

"Those big lumpy things you do tricks on. Unfortunately you can jam your ski-pole right into your sternum if your timing's not right. I've done it. Bad idea now. Dr. Hardy says I need to 'invest' in my sternum, get it real well healed up, or it might be unstable for a long, long time. It all depends on what you do. They made a bronco-buster wait nine months."

We chat about the differences in high school sports: snow-skiing in Minnesota, water-skiing in Florida.

Suddenly he says, "You want to see it?"

"Sure."

Michael pulls up his shirt. There's a neat straight line down the middle of his chest, as if someone had run a black ballpoint pen down a ruler. There are two small puncture wounds near the bottom, from drains. I don't even see any stitches.

"Looks great," I say. No puffiness, no redness. "Where's the stitches?"

"Damned if I know." He pulls his shirt back down and smiles. "I was asleep."

"Any pills now?"

"Yeah, I have a whole bunch of pills to take. Right now they cover the bottom of a coffee cup. But some are for a month, some are for two months, so that'll taper off somewhat. Aspirin for life, they say."

We look out the window at gray skies. A few students walk purposefully across the nearly deserted campus.

"The physical therapist showed me stretches, shrugs, arm swings I'm supposed to do. When I saw Dr. Oury, he told me to take off my shirt. This turned out to be a test to see how comfortable and flexible I was after the operation. He did a bunch of checks, said I had lost eight pounds of fluid, some from my lungs, and said, 'Everything is perfectly normal' and that I could go home now. God, I loved that. *'Everything is perfectly normal.'* You have no idea how wonderful that sounds. I wasn't expecting how emotional that made me feel. I felt like I had been rescued and returned to life . . . you know, like by the Lone Ranger, who rides off into the sunset. Except that it's me who's leaving. There are more emotions in something like this than you think there's going to be."

"Oh?"

"Well, just starting with my classmates. At the reunion, I told some people I was going to have heart surgery, and it was hard for even my best friends—a premature entanglement with mortality. Some didn't know what to say at all. Some were obsessed with the date, a bit of certainty, one solid fact. Several said they'd be thinking about me on that day or praying for me—people with whom I never discussed spiritual matters before—not part of our relationship.

I liked it—don't get me wrong—but it's strange, all these other dimensions you encounter when you're going to have your heart worked on. I had friends call from far, far away. My track coach from high school called. All those things add up in your mind and your heart"—Michael grinned—"and help you feel more confident."

"Is that important?"

"Oh, yeah. When you have so much time to think, it's better to think good thoughts than bad ones. Sounds obvious, but a lot of health-care people don't seem to understand that. I mean every person you deal with, whether it's the surgeon or a secretary or an insurance person—*each one* helps set the tone. Dr. Hardy came by my room a couple of times to talk with me . . . about the surgery and just regular conversation. I don't know how long he stayed—maybe it wasn't even all that long, but he made the connection with me, and that really makes a difference. Dr. Oury has had plenty of time for me, too.

"And the whole team behind you—you need that feeling. They're all individuals, of course, but each one has a moment of truth to really affect your care, and if he blows it, it's a real loss. There's all this technology—and I welcome every bit—but you need the human context as well to give it human meaning. The intensive care nurses, for example, take really good care of you—every detail. Take my second operation . . ." He raises his eyebrows.

"I heard about that. Dr. Oury said sometimes it happens, and it's usually routine, but he hates to put the family through it, because they always think the worst."

"Yeah, that's the thing. And let me tell you how they handled it. Tony—the intensive care nurse—said they were having trouble stopping the oozing from the drains. I was still zonked and wouldn't wake up. My Dad said Dr. Oury wondered what was wrong; maybe he had nicked an artery. He was real up front about it. So they wheeled me back out to the OR—and it was fast. They were not 'walking quietly.' Fifteen minutes later they sent a nurse back to my parents to say no problem, a bleeder which they'd caught and fixed. And that relieved them a whole bunch, of course."

"I'll bet," I say. "I remember when a nurse popped out of the OR to tell me that my wife Nancy didn't have cancer. Not to mention that she was obviously still alive and that everything was going routinely. If you don't know, you always imagine the worst."

"Yeah . . . and faced with the worst, you come around to what's really important. When they were bringing me out after the second operation, they were talking to me, asking me how I felt. I motioned like handwriting, and they gave me a pen and something to write on. I couldn't see because my eyes were taped shut, and I sure as hell couldn't talk, because I had a tube in my throat. I felt the paper and scribbled I LOVE YOU as best I could. I heard my Mom say she couldn't understand, so I tried again. It's not all that easy writing when you can't see or can barely keep your thoughts straight. So I tried to write TOO SLEEPY. I think they got that, but they had me stop because they could see on the monitor that my blood pressure was going up."

"You were still out of it when I dropped by. Your mom said, 'Wake up, Michael. Howard's here to interview you.'"

"She did, huh?" Michael laughs. "She got in a dig on both of us, then."

"Yeah, and I imagined that she was feeling a whole lot better."

"Yeah. That's right. By the way, Dr. Hardy watched the whole operation. He said it was absolutely textbook right through. They're thinking about using it as a teaching video. But even perfection can have flaws, like that bleeder. He said the valves were set in just right for the long term."

I ask what it's been like back at the motel.

"I had some strange dreams for a couple of nights, being spread-eagled, all stretched out. Those faded pretty quickly though. Oh, we've just been hanging out, watching some videos, talking. It's been really good." He pauses then chuckles. "One weird thing: we watched *Something About Mary,* you know that crazy, funny movie? Well, remember the part when they're trying to restart the dog's heart? I was laughing so hard I was afraid I was going to pop something, maybe even a *valve,* and my heart pillow was across the room."

"Heart pillow?"

"They give you a pillow to hold against your incision when you cough or sneeze, so it doesn't hurt so much. Well, here we were, laughing like crazy, and I couldn't reach the heart pillow or the damn remote. And then I started laughing even harder because my father, who was also cackling away, kept gasping out, 'You can't laugh! You can't laugh!' And I kept gasping, 'I know, I know!' The next day I was extremely sore, but it was worth it."

We suck on our drinks.

"Getting out of the hospital is strange; everything there is managed for you. All of a sudden you're on your own again, even if you have the help of your parents. Someone told me to bring shirts that button, since they're easier. But some things you just don't expect."

"Such as?"

"I went to the barbershop and there was a big, heavy door. I knew it was beyond what I could do. The barber stared at me as if I was weird but opened the door for me. Before he could say anything I said, 'I just had heart surgery three days ago.' And he was nice, generally speaking, although he gave me this bad-ass haircut." Michael runs his hand over his black, now short hair.

He continues. "You want to have something to signal that you're running at half speed—a sling, or a cane, or something."

I'm wrestling with a blockage in my straw. I pull it out and find a chunk of banana impaled on the end.

"Now about John Glenn . . . he was going up just as I was . . . going down, so to speak. But I thought about that: we were both facing turning points in our lives, closing one chapter and opening another. For me it's the end of the first act and the beginning of the second. Three times twenty-eight is eighty-four, my life expectancy, so this would be one-third of the way through." (Holy moly, I think. I'm almost fifty-six, twice his age, and two-thirds of the way toward this magical goal. Do I really have only twenty-eight years left?)

"I thought you were twenty-seven."

"I was. Today's my birthday."

"What? Happy birthday!" We clunk our health drinks together.

"So both mathematically and spiritually, I'm turning a page to the second act."

"Complications ensue, if I remember the standard dramatic theories."

"Bring them on." He smiles. "But going back to John Glenn. The other thing we had in common is this: we were undertaking huge adventures, relying on a lot of technology. We trusted our lives to all kinds of dials and circuits and machines, not to mention all the people running them." He pauses. "They said mortality for my operation was 6 to 8 percent."

"No kidding." Although I had wondered about this grim topic, I hadn't wanted to bring it up. "That's more than one out of twenty."

"Yeah . . . probably less for me, a young person, but if it's you who dies, that's 100 percent. That's why the support of all the medical people is so important." He pauses. "Did I tell you about the dinner?"

"No."

"Well, before my surgery my mother and my father and I all went to the Depot to eat. You know that place?"

I nod yes. It's one of Missoula's interesting restaurants, housed in a former train station.

"Well, we're having this really good meal and my mom asks me what I want done if I die during this surgery. Wow. What a question! I mean, we all stopped eating and kind of looked in each others' eyes."

Mike pauses and swallows.

"I had actually thought about this, but it's not something that's easy to bring up. My mom's a nurse, though, and she's dealt with all kinds of health issues, including death. Anyway, I had thought about it and was glad to say something. I said, if I died, I wanted my ashes spread over a lake in Minnesota. It's a lake where we used to go in the summers, and it symbolizes my childhood and all that. I also said I didn't want one of those gloomy indoor funerals, that I wanted my funeral along the same lake, but my mom said that would be too impractical because it's in too remote a spot—too far away for folks to drive to. So then I said I wanted the service to be on a hill at my elementary school that overlooks the valley and neighborhood I grew up in and my high school. It was so weird. I mean, you're supposed to take care of your parents in their old age, right? But here they're talking with me about the possibility of *my* death.

"By now all three of us are crying, right out there in the middle of the restaurant. I mean people are looking over from other tables and then looking away quickly, but it's really good. We're closer than ever before. My dad says to me the kinds of things any son wants to hear from his father. It's a hell of a thing to have to have heart surgery to get this close . . . but it's worth it. You know how it is between parents and children . . . we've butted heads before"—he brings his fists together—"over various things, how my career should go, and so on, but now our relationship is deeper than ever."

The Most Positive Attitude Going In

Michael said he liked the office of James H. Oury, M.D., because in it there were signs of intelligence and activity. Sure enough, as I enter, I see the pictures he mentioned of family, people on horseback, and Mt. Kilimanjaro. Dr. Oury gets up from his desk; he's wearing green scrubs. We shake hands. He has soft yet lively brown eyes. As we sit down at a conference table, I see Mt. Jumbo through the window behind him. I ask him about the map on his wall that shows a volcano from above.

"I took my oldest boy to climb Mt. Kilimanjaro when he graduated from high school. He thought it was such a good idea, he recommended it to the younger ones."

"How many more?"

"Two more boys and a girl."

"You've climbed it four times then?"

Dr. Oury nods. He's interested in endurance athletics both for himself and his patients.

I ask him why he has specialized in cardiac surgery.

"For me, the heart is the engine, the center of things. When you work on it you make a difference, and you know this immediately. If you work on bone or gut, you may not know for days or weeks, but with the heart, you can measure its output right away. The heart is intensely rewarding and technically challenging."

"And Michael's heart?"

"Did great. He can move all the blood he needs to at rest and during maximal activity. At rest this might be eight liters a minute, give or take—that's high normal, which figures, since he's an athlete."

"How can you tell?"

"Transesophageal echo. We do it right there in the OR. Running full out, he can now pump over twenty liters a minute. Elite athletes have been tested even higher—one swimmer was measured at fifty-four liters a minute! You can't get that with a mechanical valve, which will do fine at rest, but restrictive at the top end. That's why the Ross procedure is so exciting for me, and especially attractive to athletes."

Dr. Oury numbers among his patients a competitive kayaker, a competitive bullrider, and a mountain bike champion. "I love getting these people back to normal so they can be *active*," he says forcefully.

"We've taken Ross athletes and matched them against the local triathlon team, exercising them to exhaustion. The hemodynamics were the same. Michael's heart is expanded at the left ventricle now because it's been compensating for the valve leakage, working harder to move blood on through. After the new valve is there a while the heart will remodel to the heart of an endurance athlete."

"What was wrong with the valve?"

"We had three candidates: destruction of the valve by bacteria, calcium build-up, and congenital malformation, which was what it turned out to be. It was a bicuspid valve instead of tricuspid, but it worked well for twenty-six years. Once we got in there, Dr. Duran studied the valve to see if we could repair it. In fact, we cut through the raphe to make it tricuspid, but it would have needed stabilization that might need repair later—another operation. So Dr. Duran assisted me in the Ross procedure. Better one operation than two; Rosses run 80 to 85 percent in lasting for the patient's lifetime."

I mention how the Currys made the choice to come to Missoula.

"The technical side is very important, but so is the personal side. We like our patients and their families to have the most positive attitude possible going in. They're more fun to work with and we get better results."

"How's mortality?"

"Mortality for Rosses overall is about 4 percent. We haven't lost anybody here."

"How come Michael doesn't have any stitches showing?"

"I use a mattress stitch back and forth just under the skin." His hand draws esses in the air. "The suture material is absorbable. Since his chest is what people will see forever, I make it as neat as possible. No intern closes for me."

I ask him about the bleeder.

"We get those once in a while, but the repair is usually routine."

"How did you know it was bleeding?"

"Through the drains; the nurse kept track of the amount of blood coming out. Sometimes bleeds resolve by themselves, but with the thinners for the heart-lung machine, sometimes they don't. So we went back in, found it right away, and fixed it. I think one of the wire sutures for the sternal closure nicked the small artery that was leaking."

"And the valve placement?"

"We're very pleased: it looks just right. We videotape all our operations; we may use this one as a teaching tape. You have to get the valve position just right … it's a beautifully delicate valve, but intolerant of inappropriate stresses. You want to get it just right."

A few days later I send Dr. Oury a note, asking about a few details. I also ask about something larger: the possible role of spiritual matters. Why was I too shy to bring this up in our meeting? Or did I feel I needed all the basic things first before moving "up"?

Dr. Oury responded in writing: "Prayer and faith in God, yourself, the patient all play a part in what I do as a surgeon. I think an all-too-common perception is that we [surgeons] think we are gods. We of course are not, but the ground we tread on, the arena in which we perform, *is* hallowed ground."

And, when I sent him Michael's story for his review, Dr. Oury wrote back: "I think as surgeons—and perfectionists—we tend to focus on the technical aspects maybe to shield ourselves from the emotions involved. Michael's story brought this home to me. In *The Unbearable Lightness of Being* the surgeon at one point comments on the mystery of opening up another human's body to cure disease and his thought was that God never intended for man to be able to do that. I think He did, and it pleases Him."

WORDS OF LOVE

Michael's classmates mention spiritual matters. Dr. Oury does as well. Our last group of heart phrases centers on love, intimacy, generosity, and passion. I'll repeat some of the words and phrases, because they overlap with the previous group, the words of emotion, but here the emphases are less carnal, more positive, more psychological, more mystical, even spiritual. (In a later section we will look at the many uses of "heart" in the Bible.) Michael says there is a reverence for the heart. He appreciates the caring tone he finds in personnel at the institute. At the dinner at the Depot, he and his parents are closer because they have spoken of the taboo subject of death and they have spoken of their love.

Heartfelt, heartened, heart-to-heart talk, heart-warming, hearty, heartily, lighthearted , fainthearted, there's a place for you in my heart, speak/act from the heart, a heart as big as the sky (or Texas), a generous heart, cold hands but a warm heart, be still my beating heart, whatever your heart desires, to have a heart, to have one's heart in the right place, from the bottom of my heart, dear to my heart, with a heavy heart, with his heart in his mouth, I left my heart in San Francisco, my heart belongs to Daddy, sweetheart, to win the heart of, cross my heart and hope to die, I swear [with hand on heart].

As the heart is mortal, we can pledge our lives with our hands over our hearts, and we live in a culture that prizes purpose, direction, and commitment. A big, generous heart is good. But there is a wider set of meanings, not entirely rational or definable, that we also prize. Michael feels a human context when his family, his doctors, his caregivers express their concern; it gives him confidence. He feels the kindness and affirmation our language symbolizes in the heart, a vast, mystical reservoir of love and concern. Perhaps the most famous expression of this is Pascal's *"Le coeur a ses raisons que l'esprit ne connait point"* ("The heart has its reasons which the mind cannot know," *Pensées* 277), a caring wisdom that is beyond rational thought.

On to Mt. Kilimanjaro and More

The following summer, back in hot, steamy Florida, I pick up the phone and call Michael.

"How's your health?"

"Great. The left ventricle's shrunk back down, the leakage is way down, and the docs say everything looks good."

"So you went back to Missoula for a checkup?"

"Yeah, I could have done it here, but I wanted to work with the same people."

"It was February, right? Did you go skiing?"

"Sure did. It felt great except that I was out of shape. Seven months of doing nothing really slows you down."

"Any moguls?"

"Well, yes, I had to do a few."

"Spear your sternum?"

"Nope. I took them real slow, with lots of side to side instead of hammering right straight down them."

"So you're active again?"

"Yes, I've been running and working with light weights. The upper body strength took a knock. I've got to build it back up. Besides, we're in training."

"How's that?"

"My dad and I we're going to climb Mt. Kilimanjaro."

"No . . . like Dr. Oury and his kids?"

"Yes . . . my dad liked the pictures in Dr. Oury's office and the whole father-son idea. It'll be a kind of ritual for us of a renewed relationship. He's walking hard now to get in shape. He's lost thirty pounds."

"Fantastic!"

"Yeah, it's great. I'm really looking forward to it. We go in mid-August."

Not only has Michael's heart been repaired, he's rebuilding to a high performance level once again—and his father is joining him.

Coming to Terms with the Heart (First Essay)

I've lived with my heart for decades with little thought of it. It seems to emerge into consciousness only when I feel twinges in my chest or fear that my grandmother's heart disease may be a precursor for me—a bleak heritage. Heart, so defined, is a negative thing, a potential assassin, an organ that will betray me. I fear that my heart is a sort of Trojan horse, a fallible organ just waiting to crash, or even an enemy within that counts down the ticks like the grandfather's clock in the song that stops when the old man dies. As I bring these fears to consciousness, I regret that I've held a demeaning assumption that my heart, the mechanical pump, would eventually fail, a fated victim of material fatigue like any household appliance. Where did such a distressing definition—the heart as time bomb—come from? My grandmother, yes, but also my doctor and the mass media, for example melodramatic heart attacks in movies. Clearly our hearts have something to do with our mortality, but how can we best understand this unhappy fact? How can we most clearly perceive our hearts? What is the *stuff* of it, the *phusis* the physician studies?

I've seen hearts, touched them, listened to them, and eaten some deer heart; these sensuous encounters have given me some clues to the physical nature of the heart. There is a stuff of cardiac muscle and collagen matrix—the stuff that Dr. Duran and his colleagues observe, study, interpret, and speculate about. It is a physical organ of wondrous design and function. What language, what styles of perception most helpfully represent the heart and shape our relationship with it? As I think about the animals of the Rockies and their custom-designed hearts and about the human heart as a product of long evolution, I am more and more grateful for this organ in my chest. Part of me envies the directness of the visual and tactile experience of hearts that Drs. Oury and Duran work with, not only with Michael's heart, but with many other patients. Such direct biomedical perception of the heart is not possible for me, although I can appreciate it. I also admire how they move up their specialized abstraction ladders to metaphors and explanations that I can only partially grasp, without losing, it seems, some of the wider values we have found in our review of heart words and phrases.

The scientific views—echo, SPECT, liters/minute—are clear and exact, but they are also narrow, focused on specific sets of information. They strip away the wider connotative meanings that I value as a student of literature and as a writer. As I read cardiology books I see charts and graphs, the formula for cardiac index, Newtonian and non-Newtonian blood flows, the Reynolds number, wave forms, Bernoulli, Frank-Starling, continuity equations, and so on, all wonderfully useful in assessing the heart and its performance, but also so highly focused as to be abstract and, in some ways, reductive. They are metaphors of a precise and restrictive sort that find similarity between observations about the physical, pumping heart and numbers and graphs that can approximate relationships of well-defined factors, such as pressures, stroke volumes, and ejection fractions. Highly practical in diagnosis and treatment, they diverge from the heart values we saw in the heart words and phrases; they strip off emotional content, associative meanings, and other value dimensions—the delight of writers and readers. And yet scientific metaphors can be expanded by doctors, nurses, and patients through words into descriptions or narratives, as in the explanations to Michael of his echo tapes, or Doreen's sprinkler system—which we'll see in Kay's section. The doctors and nurses working with Michael have the scientific benefit of the technical readouts of his heart, but they also understand that all of their patients come with emotions and expectations, as well as a sense of their hearts as central and crucial to their lives. And so their conversations with them, by phone or in person, aim to calm the cultural hearts of their anxious patients before the scalpel begins to open their chests to reach their biological hearts. Thus in their delivery of medical practice they refute Descartes's heart as engine and C. P. Snow's two separate cultures.

From the humanistic side, my collection of words and phrases has underlined a wild and whirling set of values that are often subconscious, disembodied from our faithfully beating hearts. We still believe in true wisdom, courage, love, emotion, and the like, but we don't attach it so immediately to our hearts as did the ancients. The cultural metaphoric heart has become very fuzzy, perhaps to the point of dissolution, and the "heart values" we reviewed in our language have become rather indefinite, especially in a postmodern age of relativism, chaos, and multiculturalism. What does the heart value of "resolve" mean nowadays? To what deepest values do we commit ourselves? Or is it only to make money and move ahead in our workplaces? One of the many challenging aspects of the September 11, 2001, bombings in New York, rural Pennsylvania, and Washington, D.C., was the notion that nineteen men would give their lives for a particular cause. How many of us would do that?

With the domination of rational, scientific thought in our culture, the heart-as-a-pump metaphor has largely pushed aside the more traditional, cultural meanings of heart as home of the emotions, intuition, character, and the soul. And yet these meanings show up in our language at a ghostly level, fossils of a sort that we use without full awareness and with varying convictions in their truth. In this sense, the traditional heart is a phantom, one we don't quite believe in as we live our ordinary lives, although we still believe in some of the attributed cultural values. At the same time, our culture has trouble dealing with some of the capacities expelled, we might say, from the heart:

intuition, emotion, character, the soul. Thought has migrated to the brain, of course, taking up that space entirely. (Neurology tells us that the emotions have a home in the limbic system of the brain, but this news does not give us an image to which we can relate.)

Between these two views, the fuzzy and vague humanism and the specialized science beyond a layperson's ken, the heart often rests in benign neglect or even outright denial.

Paradoxically, it takes a threat to the heart to bring some of the traditional values to consciousness. For instance, when Michael's heart is threatened, his friends think about death and spiritual matters; Michael looks for a medical setting that has both technical excellence and human sympathy; he and his family find within themselves new resources of love. The negative path—cardiac illness and medical treatment—makes possible a positive one. Similarly I feel that I must first purge myself of fears and anxieties that cloud my perception of the heart. If denial and ignorance are my usual perspectives on the heart, threats to my heart open the way to serious considerations: by looking at sick hearts, I can begin to define healthy ones. I've watched how Dr. Oury has the optimally functioning heart as a gold standard, a goal in treatment. Cardiac debility and mortality help to define cardiac vitality. The word *hemodynamics* becomes more real to me, inviting me to see the power and durability of the human heart. My reading about animals' hearts tells me that our hearts are specialized according to our species, a custom-made organ for our own particular lives. One Montana evening I drive around a curve and see six deer crossing the road. They are in a slow trot, speeding up as they hear/see/smell my car. Suddenly they run at full speed, with no apparent change of gait, and they flow—there is really no other word—they flow over a fence and disappear into the woods beyond. They are athletes of their own sort, and comparable events happen millions of times a day throughout the animal kingdom, human beings included—the professional athletes we seen on TV, Michael Curry when he skis or runs, indeed, any of us climbing some stairs. Just to perform our daily tasks of getting dressed, walking anywhere, and using our hands in a dozen wonderful ways constitutes an athleticism no machine can (yet) match, an athleticism supported by our wonderful hearts. (Just standing up from being seated requires sophisticated blood control to the head so that we don't faint.) But somehow we see athletes, animals, and nature at large as separate from us, our cities, our travels in planes and cars, our electronic media, our houses, our financial status. Real athletes are on TV. Even the phrase "human nature" has come to mean something different from the nature around us, an apology for the worst in human thoughts and actions: "Oh, that's just human nature." What if we were to accept and celebrate our animal basis and nature—wherever encountered—as our wonderful homes? Loss of a sense of our hearts limits our motivation to care for these hearts and our sense of some of the wider meanings of nature around us. To understand our hearts as physical objects that are the ground, the root, the core of any metaphors—be they scientific or more widely cultural—is to take a first step in owning our hearts with pride and celebrating their wondrous structures and abilities.

One afternoon in Florida, I was approaching Bayfront Medical Center, wearing my volunteer's jacket. I was a pastoral care volunteer, usually serving in the Emergency Room/Trauma Center, although I spent one summer in the Cardiac Care Unit, gathering background material for this book. The hospital is on a busy corner with a four-way stop. I was crossing the street, properly in the crosswalk, when a car ran through the stop sign and zoomed right by me, inches from my chest. A few inches or a few seconds difference, and I'd have been knocked across the intersection and then wheeled directly into my own ER as a seriously injured patient. Such near misses make us joyful the rest of the day, but then habit sets in again. Renaissance scholars kept a human skull on their desks to remind them of the finitude of life. Artists from El Greco to Gabriele Leidloff have used skulls and skeletons to confront us with our inner, mortal selves. "Alas, poor Yorick." But it seems to me that the proper response to our hearts, even with their implied mortality, is not fear but gratitude.

Furthermore, I find comfort in what I see of the medical world. The many tools there for perceiving the heart, the surgical techniques, and the scientific drive to find new ways of understanding the heart are reassuring. Although none provides absolute certainty, and although any of these can fail, by and large they represent an abiding resource for me: my family, my colleagues, my fellow citizens. If my heart fails in any number of ways, there are technical resources to help me. And I see dedicated personnel in the medical world who have an understanding of both the scientific and the cultural heart. I see doctors, nurses, technicians, office personnel who understand patients' lack of technical expertise as well as their fears, even their terror at threats of debility and death.

Can the heart ever be known absolutely, directly, with no mediating concepts, numbers, terms? Such knowledge is the realm of the mystic, the shaman, the guru who sees holiness directly, who traffics between two worlds of the beyond and the here-and-now. I think something like that happened for me briefly in London, some twenty years ago, when Nancy and I spent a weekend in a human-potential seminar. The participants escaped from the noisy, exciting city as we gave our minds to new ways of perceiving and sharing. Our leader taught us various ways of perceiving body energy, including sensing our chakras and feeling our auras. I remember a long meditation on the heart, during which I could hear and feel each beat of my heart, even at rest; I could picture beautiful red puffs of blood rhythmically emerging from the scarlet flower in the middle of my chest. As group members shared their visions, there was enough overlap among them to understand why Hindus see chakras—seven energy wheels up the body's midline, from the anus to above the top of the head—as true representations of our energy with the same degree of certainty that we give to EKGs and echocardiograms. For Hindus, however, there's a supernatural power in this organization that we, in hospitals and clinics, have largely stripped from the heart.

What is the heart? The heart is many things, depending on who is looking at it and for what purpose. In one sense, the heart is a Rorschach test, an image that the reader interprets through his or her built-in lenses. Some of the lenses are branches of advanced knowledge. Biology, for example, defines the heart as an organ of extraordinary synthesis, as it works with blood vessels, blood, lymph, the lungs, gut, endocrine glands, the brain, even the brain's emotions and thoughts—virtually everything, we might conclude. Although enclosed in our chests—indeed well protected by spine, ribs, and sternum—the heart participates in the efforts of our footsteps, in the air of the world, and even in the emotions brought to our minds as our five senses experience the world. Sometimes called "applied biology," medicine has well exploited the metaphor of the heart as a pump to understand the practicalities of its work. (In his 1976 work, *Medical Nemesis*, Ivan Ilyich criticized such "medicalization" as a removal from human experience.) Medicine uses various technologies to assess aspects of the heart (the stethoscope for heart sounds, a cuff for blood pressure, chemical analysis for cardiac enzymes, EKGs for electrical activity). Each method of inquiry asks a particular kind of question and, given its nature, creates a particular kind of answer. Some of these—X-rays, for example—are more suited to showing structure. Others—such as transesophageal ultrasound—are better at showing function; cardiologists must assemble these various perspectives into a synthetic model for each patient, ever seeking the best diagnosis. For their part, heart patients live in their own varied worlds of fear, stress, hope, with wide variations among them in understanding medical models, as well as in motivation and ability to follow what the doctor is saying. This conversation between a doctor and a patient often tests the doctor's ability to interpret technical information to a variety of patients; appropriately, the original Latin root for the word "doctor" indicates "one who teaches." Heart surgery, less than a century old, is a new field in the human repertory, one that has quickly grown to tremendous sophistication. While watching the videotape of Dr. Oury performing the Ross procedure, I'm amazed at the opened heart within a neat border of green cloths, strangely beautiful gore under control. Heart surgery has a definiteness and a decisiveness all of its own. When Michael's aortic valve comes out and is judged finished, it *is finished*. But the heart has a durability, even under such an attack, and for Dr. Oury—as for Michael—the organ is not a machine; it is organic, active. Furthermore, the heart remodels itself after surgery, resuming the most advantageous shape once the valve is restored. Thus the heart carries an autosurgical capacity, its own innate wisdom.

The cultural wisdom of the heart, although lost to much of our conscious thought, is nonetheless an enduring gift, a way of perceiving the heart and rejoicing in it. While the Currys appreciated the technical expertise of the International Heart Institute of Montana, they also appreciated the social skills of the staff in presenting information clearly, caring for their needs, and helping them maintain confidence—human interactions rich in heartedness. Clearly the cultural heart is not dead, as we have seen in the collection of words and phrases. Center, essence, wisdom, true knowledge, home of the soul, courage, resolve, passion, love, intimacy, generosity, emotion, eros—all these have been symbolized in the heart, and these qualities are central to what it means to be a living human. As Michael said, "The heart has a special reverence"; he was proud to have a heart emblem on his hospital gown. Heart surgery allowed him and his parents, him and his classmates, even him and me (a total stranger) to become closer, open to each other. We may have forgotten the literal base of the words and phrases using "heart," but our interest in the meanings connected with it has not faded; courage, love, and wisdom are certainly prized today, but science, intellectualism, and irony have overshadowed any direct link with the physical heart. Popular culture (and we'll look at a romance novel later) has, however, kept a more naive, unexamined linkage.

Stories that use heart symbolism have power for us as models, as guides. Michael drew comfort from Arnold Schwarzenegger and Jesse Sapolu, athletes who had gone before him into Ross surgery. They are survivors of trips to the underworld, like Odysseus, Aeneas, Dante, or heroes of the mythic, night-sea journey, like Gilgamesh, Job, and Jonah. As the old spiritual has it, "Didn't my lord deliver Daniel? Then why not every man?" One of the reasons I followed Michael's surgery was, I suppose, to see whether it would work and whether he'd be returned from the stoppage of his heart to full vitality. Medical science has pursued the heart's meaning with wonderful zeal—a search for the Holy Grail, as Dr. Duran put it—but who is to care for the cultural sense of the heart, now in amnesiac disarray?

Back home in Florida, I took my stethoscope to a weekend potluck of good friends. Six of us swam in a backyard pool, ate, drank, and made jokes during a July afternoon and evening. One woman asked about my pink rectangular box, and I explained my heart project. After dinner we took turns listening to our own hearts and to each others'. People listening went into a kind of trance, their eyes closed, their lips in a slow smile. The room got quiet. We made comments about whose was faster, whose slower, hearing some differences and still, at the same time, grasping a commonality in these vital organs. This much I expected. What came next I didn't expect, although it makes sense to me now. Our conversation shifted rather sharply from the earlier companionable goofiness and hilarity of an escapist party to a meditative discussion of our parents' illnesses or deaths, people who had died recently, and friends who had died young, as if hearing our innermost pulses not only celebrated life but also invited us to consider its ultimate, mortal limits.

Did we hear ancient echoes of our mothers' hearts when we were in the womb? Many women carry their babies in their left arms, not just because they're right-handed, but because babies are calmed by hearing the maternal heart beat, which they heard for nine months at sixty-five decibels (by one estimate), the sound of a passing train. Puppies just weaned are often given a loud-ticking alarm clock to comfort them and to keep them quiet during the night. The beat of music—whether rock, country western, or classical—gives a pulse, a rhythm we instinctively enjoy.

A moment of quiet and focused attention can be restful and clarifying, whether we are listening to music or to a human heart, but the ritual is intensified by placing a stethoscope at the center of another person's chest. The stethoscope symbolizes two human urges, the urge to explore and the urge to make sense. Linking chest and ear is a decisive act, an exploration, a search into another person's inner space. The listening, however, is a different kind of inquiry, another state of being, a reception of stimuli coming toward the observer. Another version of this reaching out and receiving is the technology of the ultrasound. The ultrasound's transducer—whether the instrument on a patient's chest or a set of crystals implanted into a sheep's heart—sends out signals and then receives them. Or we might say that there's the centrifugal outward search and the centripetal inward reflection. The active and the passive, the yang and the yin, the male and the female—numerous traditions have versions of this complementary polarity, and both parts are very necessary and very human. As William Blake put it, "without Contraries there is no progression" (*The Marriage of Heaven and Hell*).

Nancy wrote a book about the alternation of action and meditation, *Martha, Mary, and Jesus: Weaving Action and Contemplation in Daily Life,* and she and I have often talked about these two poles of being. Michael Curry, our valve patient, left the active world of athleticism for the pharmaceutical hibernation of the operating room. This choice gave him, his fellow alums, and his family a chance to think about some of life's deeper meanings. During the dinner at the Depot, the Curry family faced his possible death and acknowledged in explicit words their mutual love. The realm Michael called "walking quietly" is the realm of reflection, speculation, quiet discovery, a realm of "getting heart." As a culture, we often stress the systole, the beat of the heart, its muscular effort. But the diastole, the non-beat is equally important. We more or less accept the need to sleep at night as a rhythm to our daily activities, but many Americans are not attuned to rest, regeneration, or healing calm, and many Americans are sleep deprived.

Michael's bicuspid valve had become stiff, unworkable, a parallel to my creaky, aching back. Surgery gave him a properly mobile valve; stretching returned my back to health. Stiffness in body, in thought, in one-dimensional values can lead to ill health. Professionals who pursue one goal at all costs, who work sixty hours a week, who seek out stress—such persons often live unhealthy lives. And still ... Dr. Duran and his team of scientists have in mind a Holy Grail of valves, a vision that motivates their scientific research. I think we need (or inescapably *have*) a drive to know, to find meaning through exploration, but we also need the opportunities to reflect and to let meaning come to us.

Michael, the former competitive runner, was struck by the phrase "walking quietly." His fellow alums mentioned spirituality only upon hearing of his heart surgery, news that made them slow down to think a moment. In the midst of all the American *doing,* sometimes it takes a shock to think about *being.* He and his family considered some of their deepest relationships only when his death was immediately possible. Considerations of the heart's sickness or health can bring us quickly to questions of mortality: how long will we be on earth, and for what purpose? As Michael pondered such questions in the hospital, he made what he called "an ICU promise" to himself: "If I ever get out of here, I am going to write seriously." Heart illness, support of professionals, family, and friends, and the enforced rest to consider his life all resulted in a pivotal moment for him, his career, his view of himself.

Based on Michael's story and my speculations about heart words and phrases, what is the heart? What small dossier can I assemble after the journey so far? First, of course, I must jettison my old metaphors of the assassin, the pump about to break, the Cartesian engine. Rather, I'm coming to understand the heart as a powerful and nuanced working structure, a dynamic organ that sends blood around our bodies with immediate and subtle changes based on the needs of our entire organism; it is a highly sophisticated organ that biology describes throughout an enormous range of life on earth, from worms to birds, from fish to bear, from crickets to humans; it is an organ that comes together in the human womb with wondrous precision, that changes its circulatory flow upon the birth of an infant, that can beat two or three billion times in the long life of a human. It is an organ of animals and of athletes—which means all of us—an organ surgeons can now work with in dramatic detail, although for less than a century—an eyeblink in the history of human time. Scientists have applied a huge vocabulary of words and numbers, of graphics and computer arrays to come to terms with the heart in highly specific and useful ways. Historically, other words have linked to the heart, suggesting that it was the symbolic home of some of our most basic values and concepts, a center for essential wisdom, courage, love, passion, emotion, the erotic. As science and medicine treated the heart as a pump, however, as rationalism pushed some of these notions aside, as materialism and secularism came to dominate our conscious lives, these qualities found no new home, no new image to keep them embodied and well focused for us. We still—especially if reminded—will honor them and celebrate them, but they don't seem to connect to our actual hearts, even through imaginative views. If we become sick, however, especially with a cardiac illness, we may revisit them and their possible home in our hearts.

Finally, what metaphor would I propose as a summary of this first inquiry into the human heart? The word is simple: gift. The heart is nature's gift to us, a fabulous organ of power, flexibility, and durability. It took millions of years to develop our hearts through the evolutionary chain; it took ninth months for each of us to have, at birth, a heart. As we mature, the heart shapes and develops with us. It's ours for life—*for life.*

Kay's Chronically Sick Heart
and Her Life with Many, Many Pills

CHRONIC ILLNESS . . . STORIES OF THE LONG RUN

In the emergency room in Florida where I volunteered, I saw many patients who suddenly entered the world of the sick because of traumatic events: a car wreck, a fall, an accident with a tool, a dog bite, a stabbing, a shooting, or a serious infection, such as appendicitis. These are termed "acute," meaning sudden, immediate, and serious; such patients are shocked that their ordinary world could be so quickly, so brutally disrupted. Their injuries or illnesses quickly become the focus of study for the ER staff; conditions are assessed and treated. The resources of radiology help doctors see which structures are still intact and which are broken. Car accident victims, for example, arrive strapped on a long spine board; they lie on this uncomfortable board until an X-ray "clears" their neck; movement for an unstable spine can cause serious injury, even paralysis. CT and MRI can show free air or free blood in the torso, both signs of damage. Doctors can see most fractures with wonderful clarity; sometimes they mark the break on the developed film with a red grease pencil—two little marks on either side of a white line in the bone. Such a diagnosis is satisfying—it is well circumscribed within the volume of the body, a secret found out, something ready for a specific and immediate treatment plan. In my daughter's X-ray, the two ends of her broken collarbone had drifted some two inches apart; the approach to put them back together was clear. If the treatment is surgical, a hand reaches into the body to fix the problem mechanically—like the valve shop image Michael Curry's father, Kevin, kept in mind.

Chronic illness, however, has many different features. *Chronic* relates to *chronology, chronicle,* even the Greek god *Kronos*—all variously indicating *time.* The onset of disease can be gradual . . . you don't really know when it began. Sometimes doctors call it "insidious," as if it had a malign will of its own. Chronic illness can be difficult to diagnose and to treat; no quick surgical fix is possible. In figuring out the story of the disease, physicians—at least at first—rely heavily on patient's stories, including their accounts of symptoms. Eventually physicians match up their collection of diagnoses (stories of illnesses, so to speak) with the information from the patient, the physical exam, and the labs to create a history and diagnosis. And then a new set of stories emerges, including treatment regimens, changes in symptoms, possible cures or management or palliation (comfort care), or even preparation to die.

A chronically ill person often has a serious dilemma to deal with over years, even decades, a condition that becomes a test of emotions, resolve, and imagination. Depression can come easily; any pain or cough might mean the disease is becoming worse, that treatment is failing; perhaps death is just around the corner. A chronically ill patient will need to find support systems, personal strategies, sources of hope, and his or her own sense of story to make sense of all the chaos. Failing these, a downward spiral is quite possible, often with skipped medications, missed medical appointments, and, for a few, even suicide.

Michael's valve problem could fit in the circle made by forefinger and thumb, but chronic illness may involve body systems pervasively; a collagen disease like lupus spreads over the whole body. Many chronic diseases, such as multiple sclerosis, depression, and chronic fatigue syndrome, are not entirely understood—their stories have not yet been fully written. Some of their activity operates at the microscopic level of nerves and cells. It's a different realm from the mechanics of thoracic surgery. While my love of structures led me to the anatomy lab, no comparable love of small, squishy stuff led me to the biochemistry lab. Fortunately, other folks, such as internists, cardiologists, and neurologists, delight in the intellectual puzzles afforded by chronic disease, and medicine, for them, means medicines, that is, pharmaceuticals, or drugs. The diseases are formidable opponents (or are these partners?) to work with, and any gains that physicians can make for their patients are gratifying to them and, of course, to the patients.

Because of its abstract nature—some invisible process within—chronic disease can be a difficult opponent/partner for patients to work with. Furthermore, patients vary in their abilities and motivations to understand the internal processes involved; some read furiously and press all health-care workers for details. Some give up and live in depression. More find a middle ground of understanding of the basic disorders that cause symptoms, and the general treatment strategy. Indeed, many chronic diseases can be lived with a long time, especially if they are well managed, both medically and psychologically; ideally, the patient and the physician (as well as all related staff) form a partnership, a team. Further, a treatable chronic disease can become the occasion for a patient to clarify his or her own life, a time for mobilizing inner and outer resources. The disease is a chance (an invitation?) to mend both body and mind. Some chronic heart patients find their newly diagnosed disease to be overwhelming, a terrible betrayal, a terrifying insult. After some time, some treatment, and perhaps some counseling, they often reach a relationship with their disease that includes calmness, thankfulness, and a new appreciation of life.

Such a person is Kay, whose story follows. She and many others become their own managers of their health, their own coaches in the blood sport of surviving a chronic disease. For them, many factors need to be coordinated: doctor visits, medications, health maintenance, social supports, and more. They have daily reminders of their illness and, beyond that, their ultimate mortality. A chronic illness can be a lot to deal with in a society that is already highly stressful. I found Kay's strategies, steadfast and imaginative, inspiring.

Kay, the Dream-robber in Her Heart, and the Angel of Yoga

Realizing that Michael illustrates acute heart disease with a surgical solution, I feel the need to talk with a patient who suffers from chronic heart disease. I call up Missoula cardiologist Dr. Joseph Knapp, who puts me in touch with Kay, one of his medical heart patients. She lives in another town and drives over to Missoula every so often for various errands and, of course, to consult with him. I describe my project to her in e-mails and phone calls and she agrees to help. I suggest lunch or tea, but she prefers something more private, so we meet at my office in the hospital one gray November day.

I'm standing out in the hall, looking for her, when a small, energetic woman with dark hair comes purposefully down the corridor. In fact, she seems so determined, I assume she's heading on past me and therefore say nothing. She says, "Are you Howard?" and we make the face-to-face connection. I hang up her coat and we sit down to chat. I thank her for making time for me and ask how she feels.

"I'm out of whack today. I think my potassium's low—that can do it. I'm just not comfortable in my body right now. Let's call it *borderline not happy*."

"Can you put potassium back into whack?"

"Oh, we try. I take pills for that, but they're hard on my stomach. There's no quick fix, believe me. And then there's the general living with absurdity, absurdity that's right inside of you. And central." She knocks her sternum with her knuckles.

"How did you get diagnosed in the first place?"

"I was short of breath all the time. I had no energy. Major blahs. The heart felt like it wasn't in rhythm. Or it beat faster, harder, without any real result. My regular doctor thought it might resolve, but then I had a cough that wouldn't go away. He thought maybe walking pneumonia but also heart trouble. So he referred me to Dr. Knapp."

"And?"

"He did a lot of tests. The X-ray alone showed that my heart was enlarged. The poor thing was trying to get bigger to get the job done. I guess the echo really clinched it: viral cardiomyopathy. 'Cardio' is heart, of course. 'Myopathy' means sick muscle. And 'viral' you know. Some damn virus had gotten into my heart muscle, made a home there, and weakened the muscle fibers, so I couldn't send blood to my lungs efficiently or to the rest of my body. Dr. Knapp started me on some drugs."

"And that helped?"

"Well, not right away. He said we'd have to tinker around with them until we found the right balance. It really took about a year to find the right combination. Now I see him twice a year for half an hour."

"How are you doing now—except for today?"

"Well, pretty good, except that I don't work out much with my buddies at the health club anymore. I still go there and do yoga, but I miss the routine I had going before."

"Can't work out?"

"They won't let me do weights anymore because of my heart. And I can't keep the same pace as they do, not to mention I never know when I'll crash in the middle of a workout. Just freeze up. No more energy. I also don't know how much energy I have for a day when I get up. I go to work and I'm glad to make it through the day. Sometimes I get home, though, and I'm totally wiped out. Another weird thing is that heart disease can put you into weird sleep patterns, and then you're short of sleep. I like the yoga, though." She pauses. "Funny thing, a chronic illness can make you a stronger person."

"How so?"

"Well, I take better care of myself physically. The yoga gives me strength and stamina. It makes me look healthier; therefore, I feel healthier. But especially, it's in how you live with the disease. If you get all depressed, it'll take you right down. Besides, you have to have a sense of humor. And take it one day at a time.

"It's not that I'm always happy, happy. I have my days of fear and anger. There are a lot of things I'd rather be doing, and a disease like this can rob you of your dreams. So you change some of your dreams. I mean, I have some really bad days. *Heart days,* I call them. I lie in bed with aches in my neck, my back, my hips. I'm out of it and just have to wait until things level out again."

"What does your doc say?"

"He says I'm 'stable.' The damage was already done, and nothing's going worse right now. I had an ejection fraction of 11 percent. With the drugs, I'm up to 28 percent, still below 48 percent, which is the low end of normal, but a heck of a lot better than 11 percent. He also says, 'You're doing fine; keep on going. Listen to your body, rest when you get tired, and so on.' It makes sense. Mostly.

"I mean, this thing about listening to your body. You can hear too much, I think. At any rate, he and I will keep this thing going as long as we can. It's hard to guess about energy, though. In the summer I seem to do better. I like the light. I think I'm borderline SAD [seasonal affective disorder] in the winter. I'm having full-spectrum lights put in at work." (Missoula can go for weeks with no direct sunlight in the winter.) "Of course, in the summer I sweat more and lose more potassium . . . there's always something to deal with.

"If I overdo it at the gym or at work, I'm shot the next day. And work. . . ." She rolls her eyes. "Work has a lot of stress right now. Possible mergers, layoffs. I shut it out of my mind when I go home at night. There's a good side to it during the day, though; it takes my mind off of my troubles and gives me focus. You know, that's a big word in all this . . . that's one reason I like the yoga: it gives focus. You focus on your breathing, your posture, your body, and some of the over-arching notions of energy and harmony. If I find I'm getting all out of breath, I can sit down, focus, breathe right, and feel my heart rate go down. I call it 'the flutterbies'—it's like too much caffeine, your insides all shaking. So I block out the world and calm down. Yoga is my angel."

We pause. I'm trying to think what to ask next when Kay says, "You know, I lost eighty-six pounds."

"What?"

"Yeah, eighty-six pounds."

"Gracious me." I look at her slight figure and can't imagine that kind of bulk. The skin on her face isn't loose. "However did you do that?" I think of my own struggles with just modest overweight.

"Very slowly. It took years to put it on, so I went slowly. It took three years."

"That's great."

"Yes, and I have a high school reunion next summer. I can hardly wait until all the beauty queens see me all slimmed down."

"Ha! When I went to my reunion, all the football studs were fat."

She laughs. "Yeah, it's the long run that counts. That's why I color my hair, too. If you look better, you feel better. I've tried different shades. They'd say at work, 'Trying another tint, Kay?' and I'd say, 'You're damn right.' My hair, my call. I think I've got it now."

"Looks good to me."

"Thanks. It costs two hundred dollars a year, and it's worth every penny. It took two years to find the right combination. I consider it part of my prescriptions . . . this one is for my mental health. That's the one thing that modern medicine doesn't seem to have together very well—you know, how a person deals with illness in her mind. Practical advice about hair-dyeing, exercise, how to deal with the bad days. I had to hire my own counselor. And you know, she didn't really do that much . . . just listened. Maybe that's the main thing. Where can you truly be listened to these days? You have to make your own package. That's why I go to rodeos."

"What?"

"Rodeos—you know, horses, bulls, roping, chariot races. All that stuff. I like it as a focus. It lifts your heart." She laughs. "Yeah, your heart. I travel around to the rodeos. I read the magazines. I follow the cumulative scores. I can tell you about Little Britches Rodeos or whatever you want. Friends go with me sometimes . . . they're not real keen on rodeos as such, but they say they love seeing me laugh. You have to find joy wherever you can find it . . . you've got to laugh and smile internally."

And her face is happy. The Cupid's bow of her upper lip is the center of a wonderful smile.

"It would be good if I could find a medical heart-patients group. The surgical patients have the Mended Hearts, and they can all talk about their operations. But us medical types . . . nothing so dramatic. No scars that you can see. On my really bad days, I can call on some friends, though. They help me through the tough times."

She pauses a minute. I wait.

"It's a real paradox. Some things you let go on, like with the yoga. Others, you have to take charge. I'm hell in a doctor's office. I interview them and let them know they're the science advisor; they have the expertise. But it's my body and my choice. I read my records; if that's not possible, I change to an office where I can read them."

"What's the story on this virus?"

"I don't know. I don't think anyone does. It's a mystery. And why it decided to live in my heart is another odd thing. It may have to do with my immune system, or a particular time I was ill."

"And the drugs?"

"You want to see the list?" She reaches in her purse and pulls out a small green folder from which she takes out a piece of paper that has five drugs written on it, their strengths, and the dosage. "Also a tranquilizer for when I get rattled. Insurance pays a good chunk for them, but they still run me a hundred to a hundred fifty dollars a month. I've tried some generics for some of them, but they don't work as well for me. I don't know exactly what they do, but I know they work, and that's the main point."

"How do you keep them all straight?"

"I have one of those trays for each day of the week. I count them all out at one shot. That means you have to have enough of them on hand all the time, when you travel, when . . . anything."

"So far so good?"

"More or less. I would never have chosen this path, but I'm willing to make the best of it as I can. Dr. Knapp says we'll keep it all rolling as long as we can. If my heart starts failing again and no drugs can do the job, then we'll have to look at transplantation. I'd need an AB positive heart, and those aren't easy to find. I'll cross that bridge if I come to it."

The Sprinkler System at the VA Hospital

Neurology, biochemistry, multiple systems intersecting in the heart—these all seem abstract to me, compared to the valves and chambers surgery deals with. The next summer, back home in St. Petersburg, Florida, I call on an old friend, Doreen Appunn, for some medical background. Doreen is a nurse whose career included a stint at the Emergency Room/Trauma Center at Bayfront Medical Center in downtown St. Petersburg. Three helicopters—as well as the usual ambulances—bring in patients, so there's a lot of action. As a long-time pastoral care volunteer there, I overlapped with Doreen for a few years. One memorable day, I helped her take a dead man (covered with a sheet) down to the morgue. He was dead when I came on at 3:00 P.M., and I don't remember the cause of death, but one way or another, his heart had stopped. We wheeled the gurney into the elevator and descended to the basement. Although they exist in all large hospitals, hospital morgues generally aren't labeled (bad for business—the standard med student joke is, "just feel for the greasy door knob.")

We rolled the gurney down the basement hallway; I would have kept on going but Doreen said, "It's right here." I had walked by the door many times, having no idea of its well-concealed role. Basements are a rarity in Florida, and some of the less glamorous services in hospitals are routinely put there: sterile processing, maintenance, laundries, print shops. And morgues. In a well-cooled and unlovely room, we transferred him—feet, then hips, then head and shoulders—to a table. Then we went about the awkward business of putting him in a body bag. Someone had already closed his eyes. Doreen and I didn't say much at the time, but such a shared task bonds humans who are still alive. Doreen moved on to the local Veterans Administration Medical Center (Bay Pines), where her assignment is heart research, including a stint as cardiac transplant coordinator.

I drive out to see her early one morning. The rising sun floods her office with warm light. She sits at her desk, in rose-colored scrubs. I ask about her patients in this specialized department.

"When patients are sent to us, they are usually on full medical therapy already and have very bad hearts. They are preoccupied with questions of 'When am I going to die?' and 'How am I going to die?' I can see the fright in their eyes. They want me to say, 'we have this new wonder drug that may cure your heart disease,' but this isn't, of course, the case.

"So I focus on education. If we can get a vet to know why he is taking each pill, he's more likely to take them. Better medication leads to better health, which leads to more motivation to stay well. One of our recent studies showed we have a 90 percent survival compared to 50 to 60 percent survival in the literature, and a 73 percent reduction in hospitalizations. That's what education and support can do. I give them my home phone number. I have them bring in all their meds, prescribed and over-the-counter. Some are doing herbs—which can have interactions. One man brought four big boxes of his meds; we needed a wheel chair to haul them from his car."

Grabbing a sheet of paper, Doreen says, "Here's how I explain it to lots of our patients. Many of them have high school educations or less, and they just don't grasp the different systems that interact in the heart. Some can't even read; I've had to read consent forms out loud to them. And they often confuse where the cause of illness lies and what treatments are for what problems. But we're in Florida, and they all know about lawns and sprinkler systems."

"Okay," she says, starting to sketch rapidly, "the heart is the pump, right? It lies at the center and sends water—that is, blood—out into the pipes that take care of all the lawn—that is, the body. What runs the pump? Electricity—so we'll draw that in. If the heart has arrhythmias, it's an electrical problem, which is to say, an EKG will assess the problem. Clear? Okay, where does the water or blood come from? It's city water or from the water table or, in the human, from the veins." She adds a suggestion of veins. "And where does the water—blood—go? Out into the PVC pipes to the lawn, or the arteries." She draws a branching network. (Doreen lowers her voice to say, "We're leaving out the obvious fact that blood returns back through the vascular bed.") She then resumes in her teaching voice: "If you break off some sprinkler heads, you have a bad leak, a hemorrhage, and you lose pressure in the whole system. If the leak is in the brain, you have a stroke, with damage from pressure within the skull, or you can have another kind of stroke, a clot, which cuts off the water supply to the sprinkler and part of the grass dies—that is, part of the brain. So I tell them this is bad news because too much water or not enough water can ruin a plant. Or let's say the pipes silt up and create a back pressure. What happens? The pump has to work harder to overcome this and BOOM! up goes the pressure—but with no workable result. So that's why we give Lasix—a water pill—for high blood pressure, to remove some of the fluid from the system. Or you can increase the size of the pipes by taking a nitro pill or some other vasodilators, and then the pressure on the heart goes down. And then you need to get the silt out of the pipes, or squish it against the walls—which is what we do in angioplasty—or replace them, which is a CABG—a coronary artery bypass graft—of one, two, even six arteries that supply the pump, the heart itself. Many of our patients have multiple illnesses—diabetes, emphysema, high cholesterol—which can clog up our PVC pipes. Even if we mechanically take care of blockages by ballooning or stents or rotoblading, we can only do relatively larger vessels, and the more obvious blockages. Vets like to think we've reached in and fixed everything, so we have to tell them, 'We got some of it; the rest is up to you,' because heart attacks usually come from plaques or clogs that rupture, and these can be less than 50 percent obstructed, many of them too small to treat with current technology.

"And we need to avoid the silt in the first place by eating right, exercising, and so on. If the pump itself is pretty well shot, you need an auxiliary pump, or an LVAD—a left ventricular assist device—and we're just getting implantable ones now. Or if the pump is totally shot, you need a whole new pump, and we stick in a new one, which is to say, cardiac transplantation." She stops and lays her pencil on the pad. "But finding a new heart is not easy. We've had guys on LVADs for months, even over a year. They're in the hospital with a big box attached to them, waiting for a good heart. You can't just run down to Home Depot and pick up a new pump."

"And this explanation gets it across?"

"Most of the time. As I said, they all know what a sprinkler system is, especially here in Florida, and it's something that isn't frightening—which the heart, all hidden and mysterious—normally is for them. Now all this is quite approximate, of course, but it does suggest that various systems of the nerves, the blood vessels, the blood itself, even diet and behavior—all link up in the heart. It's especially useful for explaining test results—exactly what's wrong, and therefore what treatment can help them. And this helps keep them motivated to come for appointments, to take their meds, to do their rehab—whatever they need.

"A lot of vets have seen hard times, in the service and elsewhere. A lot of them are blue collar. Some have wounds and illnesses from being in wars. Many smoke." (The lung service at most VA hospitals is usually huge; WWII vets were often given cigarettes provided by tobacco companies. With little other rewards, cigarettes became widely used "over there," and vets came back home with the eventual problems—now predictable—of lung cancer and emphysema.) "Some have mental problems. Some have drug and alcohol problems. Some have been kicked around. So sometimes it's hard to get many of them excited about what they can do to get well and stay well. If they understand, even at the most basic level, something about the heart, it can really help.

"Sometimes I tell them that the heart's a kind of Grand Central Station—just about everything runs through there, one way or another, and they can control a lot of those things. Some things they can't control, like their genes, but lots of other things they can, like smoking. I tell them nicotine and caffeine are vasoconstrictors, things that narrow your PVC pipes, which is bad."

Doreen's a friendly soul, and her office has its own Grand Central Station feeling. I ask whether Art Jackson, whom I know from church-music circles, might be around today. Doreen gives him a call on his pager and he joins us later in the morning. He's a tall man, a pharmacist by trade. We make small talk about his present assignment—security for scheduled drugs, such as narcotics. I ask him about heart drugs.

"Well, there's a whole flock of those, of course. What we've been especially interested in lately is the number of patients we get *because* they're taking drugs, and I mean licit drugs, regularly prescribed drugs. Ironic, no? The drugs are supposed to help, of course, but they're a leading cause of hospitalization for us."

"Why is that?"

"There are the regular side effects, and even some rare adverse reactions, but a large cause is noncompliance among the patients, especially the elderly. They forget to take them, double up when they miss, or misrepresent to us their dosage. Take a patient needing diuresis to cut the blood volume to help the heart out. I'll say, 'Are you taking your water pill?' and they'll say, 'Oh yes,' but it turns out they've cut the dose in half to stretch out the bottle for economic reasons. Or they're going on a car trip, and they don't want to stop for the bathroom, so they skip the pill and then run into trouble. And, again for older folks, it just gets complicated. They've got a chart a foot thick; they're on thirteen different medications; they've got insurance hassles, and on and on. It's a lot to deal with when you're old and tired."

John Lebel stops by and sits down. He greets Doreen warmly. He's a cheerful, relaxed man of about sixty, I'd guess. Rebecca, another heart research nurse, joins us, greeting John fondly. She starts to tell me the story.

"John here is one of our transplants. We're so proud of him. Doreen was the transplant coordinator." Doreen smiles.

As if a baton has been passed, he picks up, "Yeah, I went home to die until these research people got hold of me." I sense a remarkable bond between him and these two women; they have helped to save his life—twice, it turns out: first, by helping him get a new heart, and, second, helping him through what appeared to be a rejection crisis. He and Rebecca tell the story of his second trip to Richmond, Virginia, where the McGuire VA Center had done his transplant. It's a common text they all share. They finish each other's sentences and prompt each other for further details. Rebecca begins.

"He looked terrible."

"I just wasn't feeling good."

"We got lab results back that looked kind of scary."

"I had gone to lunch."

"And we couldn't find him right off. Even with his beeper."

"Turns out I was right here in the hospital."

"Doreen said, 'Do you have any gas in your car?' Fortunately, I had just filled up."

Doreen adds, "I called over to the airport and had the tickets waiting. We had the plane wait, too."

"Rebecca grabbed me right out of my lunch."

"I didn't have time to phone anyone or let him pack."

"No luggage, no pajamas, no toothbrush," John says.

"We made it in twenty minutes." Thinking over the route, I'd have figured forty minutes, minimum.

"Amazingly enough, there was a parking place right by the elevator. But how was I to find a wheelchair?"

"And there was one right there—must have been divine intervention," John adds.

"We got on the plane just before they closed the door."

"And it was a very bumpy flight."

"We were afraid of being diverted to another airport, another state. We'd miss the rendezvous!"

"But we landed in Richmond all right, and they grabbed us right off the plane."

"And whisked us over to the hospital."

"All his records were already there."

"They did a right heart cath and biopsy right away."

"It wasn't really rejection, but he needed to have his drugs adjusted."

"And then we came back. So here I am. I'm on three drugs."

"He's doing great."

"I feel good. And I'm so damn grateful to everyone . . . to this team. And, of course, to the family that allowed me to get this heart." He pauses. "The donor was a twenty-three-year-old man who died in a motorcycle wreck. I wanted to send the family a note of thanks, but that's kept confidential."

BEYOND THE PUMP AND SPRINKLER SYSTEM

Doreen's sprinkler system metaphor is a good one for her audience, and roughly accurate as far as it goes. It's limited to the major systems of the body, of course, and it's largely a mechanical illustration to help the vets understand the cardiac information by matching it with images vets already know. Throughout the Montana fall, I've been reading in cardiology journals and books about more elaborate models, typically expressed in biochemical language of forbidding complexity. Luckily, when I travel to Houston, Texas, for a meeting of the American Society for Bioethics and Humanities, I share a cab from the airport with a doctor who can interpret some of the details. Gary Grant, M.D., is an internal medicine doctor from Pacific Grove, California, where he does a lot of cardiology. A former athlete, he is now the doctor for his son's high school football team, pacing the sidelines and closely observing the game. When I ask him about sports injuries, he says, "If you can see exactly how a kid gets banged up, you're already ahead in knowing what damage to look for." I ask him if he might have time during the meeting to help me with cardiac neurohumoral arcana, and he says, "Sure." Two days later we have supper on the first floor of the Galleria, overlooking the ice rink where Tara Lipinski used to practice. I have a list of questions to which he responds excitedly. I can tell he loves the heart and everything that links to it.

"We keep learning more and more about the brain's relationship to the heart—this is a huge concept," Gary says over our salads. "Biologically speaking, the heart is relatively stupid, that is, passive. It does what hormones and nervous impulses tell it to do.

"Let's start with the autonomic nervous system, the one that runs your heart and inner organs—as opposed to the peripheral nerves that run all the muscles and signal hurt if you stub your toe. The autonomic nerves are an inner system, so to speak, and there are two branches, the sympathetic and the parasympathetic. Basically, the sympathetic branch serves to activate or jazz up. This is important for any emergency—the old fright/fight/flight syndrome. My football players are doing a lot of this. The parasympathetic branch, naturally, does the opposite: slows down, relaxes, mellows out. That would be—or should be—for study hall or digesting hamburgers. The nerves of the heart run through the SA node—the sinoatrial node—a kind of control center for cardiac impulses. There are substations called bundles of His, named after the

Swiss physician Wilhelm His Jr., and further branchings to, eventually, every cardiac muscle cell. If this sequencing gets messed up, arrhythmias occur and the heart doesn't pump right. Sometimes we shock people's hearts—cardiovert them—to put the electrical system back to zero, so to speak, so it can start working right again. Or we use drugs. Or ablation."

"What's that?"

"We go in with a wire and fry the misbehaving cells. It's really ingenious: you snake up from a puncture in the groin artery to the heart and zap them in precise locations from the inside of the heart. Then all the behaving cells can work together correctly again. Some of the bad guys are easy to find, but some are difficult. You may have to try several times. Or maybe never find them. In some of this work we're on the edge, with no guarantees. But when it works, it's fabulous. We can take patients off most of their medications."

"How does the SA node know what to do?"

"We don't really know, but it's born with a certain metronomelike rhythmicity; beyond that, it accepts messages from nerves and hormones to raise and lower its rate. The heart muscles are set at something like forty beats per minute forever. They'll beat for a while even in a dead body without an SA node, but not in a very productive way. They'll even beat outside a body for some hours in, say, a saline solution. Talk about persistent."

"Yeah, I've seen that on film of a heart transplant. They take out the old one and put it in a stainless steel pan, where it tries to beat all by itself."

"Totally weird, but good for us when hooked up right so that the muscle works faster, some seventy beats per minute at rest and higher, of course, under loads."

"And all that's hardwired?"

"So to speak, but it's more complex than that, since it's interactive and at microscopic levels. You couldn't just give it to an electrical engineer to replicate."

"OK, so what's neurohumoral?"

"*Neuro* is nerve, of course. *Humoral* means liquid. You could think of it as a liquid connection for biochemical agents within and between cells and the entire bloodstream. This is truly amazing stuff, very subtle controlling messages, a whole series of analog adjustments in contrast to some kind of digital nerve hookups—if you don't mind a little computer language. These are functioning in you and me right now and, of course, all the time. It's only when they are out of synch that medicine is called on to figure out why and what to do."

"OK, so there's a link between the nerves and the humors, or liquids, which really mean hormones and ions, basically?"

"And neurotransmitters. It's miraculous ... truly the beauty of physiology," he says. I'm worried he won't finish his supper because he's talking a mile a minute.

"In the sympathetic branch of nerves, there are two kinds of activation, called alpha and beta." Gary writes the Greek letters on a napkin. "You've heard of beta-blockers? That means a drug blocks the connection at the beta receptors in the heart muscle. There are millions of these all over your body, and particularly in the heart, which we can target with drugs. Cardiac tissue has thousands of little switches in the muscle fibers called receptors; they turn on or activate when the right hormone touches them. A sick heart needs to be protected against running too fast or too strongly, so we give beta-blockers, which block the action of epinephrine—adrenaline—at, obviously, the beta sites. A healthy heart needs these hormones to jump right in and stimulate the heart to respond to a workload. And there are two systems affecting these receptors' work, adrenergic and cholinergic. The -*ergic* part of the word means work, like *ergonomics*. *Adren* is for adrenaline, and the *cholin* is for acetylcholine. For a beta-adrenergic site, the adrenaline would hit it, turn it on, and excite action. Thus if you slow down this point of stimulation, you can lower heart rate, and you can relax tension in the blood vessels, making blood pressure fall. Both are good in heart patients who need less of a load on their hearts."

"Whew," I say, writing frantically. "This is complicated."

"Yeah, it is. That's what's fun when you're trying to help a patient, trying to apply knowledge and improve function with medication. I get a kick out of explaining it to patients too. It's a big complicated picture of interacting forces and you have to find the right buttons to push. Also, it's more complicated than I'm telling you."

"The big picture is all I need."

"All right, the alpha receptors constrict the fine muscles along blood vessels, thereby raising vascular resistance and blood pressure. They're triggered by norepinephrine and epinephrine. These adrenergic humors help prevent us from going into shock all the time, for example, when we stand up quickly.

"The whole cardiac system is a series of feedback loops. Baroreceptors are cells that register pressure, you know, like in the word 'barometer.' These lie at spots along the vasculature and can register if blood pressure is falling too low, which would be dangerous for the brain, the kidneys, and so forth. The baroreceptors, in such a case, signal to the brain to signal to the hypothalamus to release vasopressin from the pituitary gland which will work with the adrenal hormones to constrict the arterioles to raise blood pressure. We can mimic that process with drugs when the body's system isn't doing that to the level we need. Vasopressin is also used as a drug that's given to bleeders, for example, to help tighten up their blood system. Or we can give something called an ACE inhibitor, which blocks the angiotensin-converting enzyme that drives the production of angiotensin, which—as the name indicates—constricts blood vessels and therefore raises blood pressure. So an inhibitor of this mechanism would lower blood pressure. And then there's Lasix . . . you've heard of it?"

"Yeah, they give it to racehorses."

"That's right . . . for the same reason as to humans. It's a diuretic, which makes you pee, which removes water from your blood, which means that your blood volume decreases, which means the heart is working with a smaller load to move, which means it can work easier and better. Or maybe you want to make the peripheral vasculature space bigger to help the heart out, then you give calcium-channel blockers to block the innervation of tiny muscles constricting vessels. It's a series of balancing acts, with trade-offs no matter what you do, which is why you have to keep getting feedback from the patient. It's tricky. And fun."

"We're talking ions, here, right?"

"Yeah. The sarcolemma, which is a system of invaginations off the surface membrane of the heart muscle cells, has little channels through which the basic ions—sodium, potassium, and calcium—can go. It's really amazing: we're talking small amounts of shift here, and over and over, with the speed of each heartbeat. By letting these ions in and out, the cells create the electrical forces that allow the cells to fire, that is, to contract. If your potassium is too low—hypokalemia—your muscles get weak." (I think of Kay back in Montana.) "If this continues, they paralyze. Further still, you die. Or too much potassium will do it too. For executions, potassium chloride is given by injection, along with a tranquilizer and a muscle relaxant. It stops the heart muscle, and BANG you're dead.

"The heart can be considered a mechanical pump, taking in and shooting out blood—sure—but it's also a *chemical* pump as well, and there's got to be the right balance or you're messed up. If you have too much sodium, you'll have too much blood, because water follows sodium. And the result is volume overload, or what we call congestive heart failure. The heart can't keep up with the blood coming into it; the blood backs up into the lungs, and the lungs get wet and congested: pulmonary edema. You cough . . . sometimes pink fluffy stuff comes out of the mouth. It's hard to breathe, because the patient is drowning in his own fluids."

"Yeah, I've seen that in the ER. It's really alarming."

"It looks terrible, but it's often easily fixed with the right drugs. Some Lasix opens up the kidneys and blood vessels and nitro opens up the peripheral veins so that the blood volume is held back from the heart to unload it, so that it can recover. Since sodium and water go together, and Lasix sends sodium out through the kidneys and makes you pee, the volume overload drops, the lungs clear up, and things get a whole lot better. Ordinarily the brain and the kidneys talk to each other to keep the balance right. The kidneys can hold back water with sodium or let it all go to the bladder. Thus the heart is the benefactor of normal kidney function. And once again, everything links up."

"So you can really help people."

"Definitely. We're talking about saving people's lives in the acute situation and extending people's lives in the chronic situation. If the usual dynamics of the body fail, we do our best to help with pharmacologic therapy. It's a challenge, since drugs are never perfect."

"Say some more about congestive heart failure."

"It's kind of a catch-all term for a vicious cycle, and it can happen for a number of reasons—failures in the kinds of physiologic systems we were just talking about. In CHF, for whatever reason, the heart can't pump the blood out fast enough so it backs up in the pulmonary circuit, and its pressure drives fluid through the alveoli's walls and into the lung airspace. At its worst, the patient is basically drowning in his own secretions. It gives a feeling of terror."

"Very bad news."

"Yeah, and there can be a crackling sound in the lungs—what we call 'a death rattle.' In the old days, it always meant you were finished. With today's drugs, you can often dry out the lungs and pull someone back from this terrible situation."

I check my list of questions. "What about loads?"

"Very important. If you're talking about blood coming back to the heart, it's the preload. You can decrease preload by reducing the blood volume with diuretics or by expanding the veins. Nitroglycerin is the most famous agent for expanding veins. At higher doses, however, it also expands the arteries, which carry, of course, the afterload, that is, blood coming from the heart. Some drugs routinely do both. You have to pick the right ones . . . and watch out for side effects, especially over a long term. That's one of the trickiest things about a chronic heart patient."

Like Kay, I think. We finish up our meals. We both want to cruise the four floors of stores around these strange atria. An atrium was originally an entrance way or a courtyard for a Roman house; I remember them from the ruins at Herculaneum. Now an atrium can be in a hotel, the human heart, and in the Galleria, where not blood, but expensive goods, money, and tourists are pumped through. What kind of metaphoric atria are there for a new understanding of the heart? The labs at the International Heart Institute of Montana? Doctors like Gary who can explain technical matters to laypeople? A text that touches our intellect, emotions, and spirit?

Gary offers a final comment. "The heart, whether we call it stupid or not, really knows what it's doing in the sense that all these complex systems run through it and ordinarily they work very well, usually in perfect sync. When something doesn't work, we have to figure out why and take steps to restore what's missing or work around it. The surgeons do it more mechanically; we internists do it with drugs that try to mimic what's supposed to be happening naturally. The heart can often respond very well with just a little help."

"That's great. You must like your work."

"It *is* great. And I do like my work. But there are also those inevitable times when everything we do isn't enough, and the patient gets sicker and dies."

As I fly back to Montana, I go over my notes. Gary has given me a coherent story of how the heart works at a biochemical level. He's shown me that his medical practice mimics the basic story of the heart's working with substitutions, trying to replicate the ideal heart activity—at least as we understand it so far. He knows multiple stories of ways the heart doesn't work as well, matching them up with the narratives for healing he has learned. Such are the instrumental meanings, the tools he can apply to patients' hearts. Less easy to define is another quality of his descriptions, his enthusiasm and love for the heart and his compassion for patients in distress. If my heart were failing, I'd want a doctor like him.

Hearts in Literature

In classic western literature up to the Renaissance, hearts were unifying symbols, showing connections between mind and body, thinking and feeling, even the human and the divine. After the Renaissance, the meaning of hearts divided into different realms, although sometimes these realms overlapped. The relative newcomer, science, redefined the heart as a pump, ignoring the unifying senses of the home of wisdom, intuition, the soul, the emotions; the heart was now primarily a functional group of tissues with a specific job to do: propel blood around the body. Furthermore, it could be rationally understood and, by the late twentieth century, well manipulated by drugs and surgery. Literature, however, still maintained many of the classical meanings, especially in the Romantic writers, such as Wordsworth. As industrialization, science, and rationalism marched on, however, serious writers became increasingly secular and more selective in using hearts as symbols, to the point of ambivalence and, even, irony. Folk and popular literature, on the other hand, still kept some of the classic values of hearts as the seats of intuition and emotion, while hymns and other sacred literature have maintained religious meanings.

The oldest literary work that has survived is *The Epic of Gilgamesh,* dating from the third millennium B.C.E. I don't read Sumerian, but comparing translations tells me that the word "heart" is used routinely for the Sumerian *sha.* In

N. K. Sandar's version, some sixteen references to the heart tell us what is in a character's mind and whether a man has courage or fear or compassion. When Gilgamesh and Enkidu kill the bull of heaven, they cut out its heart and offer it to the god Shamash, the heart being a symbol of life, essence, power. Enkidu "pours out his heart" to his friend, Gilgamesh. When Enkidu dies, Gilgamesh "touched his heart, but it did not beat, nor did he lift his eyes again. When Gilgamesh touched his heart it did not beat." Reading such repetition gives us a ritual sense of the death of Enkidu and of the friendship between them. While Gilgamesh journeys to the land of Faraway to learn the secrets of mortality, we read a formulaic phrase four times: "Gilgamesh feels despair in his heart." Learning that man is mortal and that there is no permanence, he laments having "wrung out his heart's blood" with his efforts. As with the ancient Hebrews (we will discuss Biblical references later), the heart is a symbol of life and vitality, but also a place of emotion, inner feeling, knowledge, and power.

Similarly, the ancient Greeks used *kardia* in several senses, including soul, mind, and the seat of vitality, as well as courage, strength, and various emotions, according to an Ancient Greek-English dictionary and my colleague Professor Gary S. Meltzer. In Homer's *Odyssey,* the word heart (in the Greek variations of *kardia, etor,* and *thymos*) occurs three times in the crucial Book 23, when Odysseus has returned and killed the suitors but still must win the trust of Penelope. In Fitzgerald's translation

> She turned then to descend the stair, her heart
> in tumult. Had she better keep her distance
> and question him, her husband? Should she run
> up to him, take his hands, kiss him now? (Book 23, ll. 85–88)

Telemachus urges her to sit with the disguised Odysseus and question him so that she can recognize and accept him. "Your heart is hard as flint and never changes!" (l. 100) he concludes. When she finally knows for sure that her husband has returned, "her knees / grew tremulous and weak, her heart failed her. / With eyes brimming tears she ran to him" (ll. 205–07). In Sophocles' *Antigone,* the word "heart" occurs several times, as characters speak of the turmoil within them, or a messenger describes it. In the Roman world, Virgil's *Aeneid* presents Dido suffering from an anxious heart (*corda oblita*) as Aeneas leaves her; soon, she kills herself.

The medieval poem Beowulf uses heart (*heort*) and its compounds in two ways. Several phrases indicate character or mood. Beowulf is greathearted (*rumheort*), stouthearted, or firm-hearted; he carries sorrow in his heart after the death of Herebeald. Even a raven is blithe-hearted. The second usage is imagery of death, revealing the heart as a vital center. In assessing his life, Beowulf recalls how he broke open the "bone-house" and "heart-streams" of an enemy. Beowulf's life will end when "death's flood" reaches his heart—an interesting reversal of the liquid imagery of blood fatally overwhelmed. It is a poem of a world with harsh realities, such as wars and monsters, but a good king has the proper heart to lead and act courageously until his death.

The medieval story of Tristan and Iseult, in many versions, uses heart for the lyric essence of the tumultuous lovers; in Bedier's version, Iseult cries out, "Oh friend . . . fold your arms round me close and strain me so that our hearts may break and our souls go free at last." Here, erotic love merges with a spiritual freedom. St. Teresa of Avila runs the trope the other way, suggesting that religious pain and joy have a sensuous dimension, as an arrow of love enters her heart. (Bernini's statue of this event emphasizes her erotic nature as she bares her breast to a Cupid-like angel who aims the arrow at her heart.) In Dante's *Divine Comedy,* the heart (*cor*) has, again, several uses. The pilgrim Dante announces the fear in his heart at the outset of the *Inferno,* while the sly Francesca of Canto V assures him that she was not at fault in adultery, because love (Amor) seized the heart of Paolo, her lover. In the *Paradiso,* Piccarda, on the other hand, maintains her purity by wearing a veil over her heart. Dante himself, his moral education nearly complete, feels that his heart can give itself to God as no mortal heart could before. As the poem moves toward its climax of religious vision, St. Benedict urges Dante to look back on earth so that his heart, in joy, can be ready to see the triumphant Christ.

Shakespeare is a prodigious user of heart words and phrases; one concordance lists over a thousand usages. According to Schmidt's *Shakespeare Lexicon,* the meanings largely overlap with today's usages (or, we could say, Shakespeare helped establish today's usages): the seat of affection or emotion; a prompter of will and inclination; the seat of love and amorous desire; the motive or activity (courage, spirit); the soul or mind in general, even the power of thinking; also the core or essence. The uses in the tragedies are typically darker than in the comedies. Macbeth acknowledges that his "false face must hide what the false heart doth know," but Bottom exclaims, "The eye of man hath not heard, the ear of man hath not seen, man's hand is not able to taste, his tongue to conceive, nor his heart to report what my dream was" in *Midsummer Night's Dream.* One emphasis that we no longer believe is the concept that a surplus of emotions can actually burst the heart, according to my colleague Professor Julienne H. Empric. In *King Lear,* for example, Edgar says, "List a brief tale; / And when 'tis told, O that my heart would burst!"

Romantic poets love the heart, a symbol of emotional richness and intuitive harmony, often with nature. Wordsworth writes, "My heart leaps up when I behold / A rainbow in the sky" and opines that poetry offers "truth . . . carried alive into the heart by passion." Keats declares, "My heart aches" in the opening line of his "Ode to a Nightingale" and refers to "the sad heart of Ruth" later in the poem. In his lush "The Eve of St. Agnes," young Porphyro comes to the castle "with heart on fire," while Madeline's "heart was voluble" (talkative). After her meditative prayers, "her heart revives," the lovers join in love, and Madeline declares, "my heart is lost in thine."

Although only a generation later than the English Romantics, Edgar Allan Poe adds another dimension that undermines many of the affirmative senses of the heart, an ironic usage of the heart as conscience in "The Tell-Tale Heart." Our deranged narrator "chuckled at heart" upon hearing the old man's groans in the night, which excite him "as a beating of a drum stimulates the soldier into courage." He fears neighbors will hear the heart or that, in Shakespearean fashion, it will burst; so he kills the man. Although he rationally hides the body, the heart beats on in his mind until he reveals to police the hiding place of the "hideous heart." Baudelaire, a devoted reader of Poe, entitles a confessional diary *Mon coeur mis à nu* (*My Heart Laid Bare*), and Flaubert outright makes fun of Emma Bovary's heart (*coeur*), "where the spider of boredom weaves its web in the shadows of every corner." It is Baudelaire, however, who offers the most negative vision in his poem "A Voyage to Cytherea" ("Un Voyage à Cythère"). In classical mythology, Cytherea was the island where Venus (Aphrodite), the goddess of love, was born from the sea. In Baudelaire's "Voyage," the speaker travels to this island where he sees a gibbet with a dead man hung upon it, rotting. Terrible birds have eaten his eyes, his testicles; his guts hang on his thighs. Below, ferocious beasts turn and prowl, their muzzles upraised. Then the terrible climax: the poet sees himself in this doomed man, an emblem not only of failed love, but of the vilest carnality. The poem closes:

> "Ah! God! Give me the strength and the courage
> To contemplate my heart and my body without disgust!"
> ("Ah! Seigneur! Donnez-moi la force et le courage
> De contempler mon coeur et mon corps sans dégoût!")

(In French, the semantic likeness of *courage* and *coeur* is clear, and the similar sounds of *contempler, coeur,* and *corps,* suggest that they all overlap—or might overlap; there is no assurance that God will grant the speaker's prayer.)

A modern temper has been established. The heart can now be suspect, a place of boredom, guilt, and pain. Conrad's *Heart of Darkness* suggests the basic animality and barbarism of humans. Graham Greene's *The Heart of the Matter* portrays singularly unhappy characters with no hope of salvation;

although, according to one critic, faith is the heart of the matter, but the novel is so dark and tragic that we might say there is no heart at all.

Although editors provided the lyric title for Carson McCuller's novel *The Heart Is a Lonely Hunter,* it well represents the book's difficult themes and images. We read of Dr. Copeland—"In his heart there was a savage violence," "the thought of each of these white men was bitter in his heart," and "his heart turned with this angry, restless love,"—and we feel the instinctual power of this novel to reveal the passions and urges of people in a poor southern town around 1940. Their turmoil with racism and sexism mirrors distant Nazi atrocities, but instances of revelation and grace are also possible. On the last page Biff has an "illumination." "His heart turned and he leaned his back against the counter for support" as he catches a glimpse of love between "bitter irony and faith." In this novel, the heart is an essence of all persons, lonely hunters in a dangerous world; it keeps an emotional record of fleeting hopes and frequent tragedies.

Popular fiction revels in heart symbolism, if Sharon Sala's *Roman's Heart* may be considered typical. This is a 1998 "Intimate Moments" book published by Silhouette Books, self-proclaimed as "America's Publisher of Contemporary Romance." In 250 pages there are some fifty mentions of hearts, heartbeats, and pulses, mostly having to do with emotions of love, lust, fear, uncertainty, and revenge. As the title indicates, many of these are attributed to our macho hero, Roman, whose armored heart slowly loosens to feel love for the heroine, Holly. We have *hammering hearts, hearts pulsing, hearts skipping beats, a knife in the heart,* and other standard phrases. The other emphasis is in phrases like "her heart told her" which suggest intuition, certainty in love, and wisdom beyond what men can know. Holly tells him, "I fell in love with you, and when we made love, it sealed that fact in my heart," echoing "set me as a seal upon thy heart" from the Bible's *Song of Songs.* But here there are no religious dimensions, no wider truths about the universe. The heart is the place of emotions and intuitive truth, a measure of passion, and a place that men keep locked up. While the heart phrases (and virtually everything else in the book) are clichés, these are clichés that sell very well to readers—mostly women—seeking guided fantasies in which passion and faithful love coincide.

The word "heart" is much beloved by writers and booksellers for marketing purposes. The Barnes & Noble Web site lists some 7,500 titles or subtitles of books with the word "heart." Some of these books are biological or medical; some are self-help books; some are religious; many are works of fiction.

Serious literature, for the most part, has abandoned any sense of the heart as a place of truth, wisdom, or religion; through irony, sarcasm, even ridicule, the traditional meanings of the heart are attacked and abandoned. If these abstractions can be entertained at all, they do not reside in the physical heart, but in the brain. And with the arrival of Freudian psychology, the unconscious mind is clearly a dangerous portion of the brain. Popular literature typically avoids the philosophical or religious dimensions, focusing on the emotional, the erotic, the intuitive. On the one hand, the physical heart is still present to show the excitement of romantic love, thus pairing physiology and mental states intimately. And yet the suggestions of intuitive knowledge and perfectly matched lovers (as in *Roman's Heart*) are idealistic to a superhuman extent. Such popular literature works as a ritual event, affirming basic wishes without reflection, analysis, or exploration of implications.

The realm of the heart in serious literature of the last 100 to 150 years becomes problematic, compared to the values associated with the heart in ancient times. The ancient meanings are positive and synthetic of human experience; they tend to be coherent among themselves so that courage, the soul, and love can all reinforce each other. In modern times, the heart—having become the pump of science, having lost thinking and feeling to the brain, having become for many authors disconnected from spiritual life—is a confused and confusing place. Small wonder it's easy not to think about hearts.

There are, however, some exceptions.

Humans seem especially interested in stories of illness and injuries (technically called "pathographies") that show some of the extremes humans may face and ways they may survive them. Some of my favorites include Oliver Sacks, *A Leg to Stand On;* Richard Selzer, *Raising the Dead;* Lawrence M. Pray, *Journey of a Diabetic;* Audre Lorde, *Cancer Journals;* Reynolds Price, *A Whole New Life;* and William Styron, *Darkness Visible.* These tales give their body-and-mind version of the night-sea journey, the archetypal myth of human journeys into the dangerous beyond, and the return with some kind of healing and/or new understanding. Some of the classical examples would include the *Epic of Gilgamesh,* the *Odyssey,* the book of Job, the book of Jonah, the Gospels, and Dante's trilogy. All of these stories—like the contemporary Schwarzenegger and Sapolu figures for Michael and the rodeo competitors for Kay—give us positive models, paradigms for human tragedy and healing: *If these other people can survive hard times, so can we.* Because they guide our imaginations through difficult realms, these are stories that heal.

A particularly fine example of such stories is Gretel Ehrlich's *A Match to the Heart* (New York: Pantheon, 1994), in which she inspects the workings of the human heart. The title of the book extends our discussion of words in Michael's section because it contains intersecting meanings, stories, and, even, puns. First, "a match" suggests simple illumination, the way we'd light a match in the dark to see something; similarly, Ehrlich inspects the workings of her heart in this book.

There may even be a reference to the largely lost notion of candling: holding an egg up to a flame to see whether an embryo has formed within. Next is the more general sense of a "match" as a pair, or a partnership, for example, the various healing pairings in the book, such as Ehrlich and her cardiologist Dr. Blaine, and also Ehrlich and her dogs, which help her to heal. Finally, we have the dramatic literal event that starts the book: Gretel Ehrlich was struck by lightning as she walked on her ranch in northern Wyoming one August afternoon, much as we'd strike a match and see it suddenly burst into flame. Puns have been called the lowest form of humor, probably because they challenge our sense that language should be efficient and one-dimensional, but Shakespeare and many other writers have used puns as a way of showing conjunctions of meaning.

Ehrlich's story includes the acute injury of the lightning strike and the aftermath (sequelae, in medical terms), a chronic neurological condition that dramatically affected her heart—and therefore her life—for over two years. Her book illustrates a powerful way words may be expanded, the linear assemblages we call stories. If words name and, to some extent, evaluate reality, they can also give suggestions of order, causality, and synthesis when they're linked into narratives, many of which become models or guides for living.

When Gretel Ehrlich was hit by lightning, the electrical energy damaged her sympathetic nervous system, the jazzing up branch Dr. Grant described. The parasympathetic system, therefore, ran unchecked, telling the heart to slow down. Thus she had little energy, low blood pressure, and a propensity for fainting. This diagnosis was arrived at with some difficulty; it comes about one quarter of the way through the book, after Ehrlich undergoes some futile treatment in rural Wyoming. In California, however, a specialist solves the mystery, and cardiologist Blaine Braniff gets her on the right track, in a partnership (or match) that expands as the book progresses and she begins to heal. When she's well enough, she accompanies Blaine on his cardiac rounds to learn more about the heart—both as a physical object and as an emotional/social/spiritual repository. Ehrlich enjoys watching how Dr. Braniff touches his patients, listens carefully, and talks openly and lovingly with them. He treats his patients as whole persons, persons whom he loves. With his help, she also observes heart surgery, reporting, "I felt as if I had broken into a hidden cave and come upon rubies and sapphires. Looking past skin, red tissue, white bone, into a chest held open by a steel frame, I saw a beating heart." She also researches the nature of lightning, attending the Third Annual Conference of Lightning Strike and Electric Shock for Survivors. In all of these researches (and there are others—Buddhist thought, biological contexts, a local Indian tribe), Ehrlich brings words to make order out of chaos, sentences to put things in line, stories with beginnings, middles, and ends.

Through this wonderful book we enter her difficult world and rise up, once again, with her. It's a ritual that recognizes tragedies all of us have already survived and offers a dress rehearsal for tragedies that are yet in our futures. Such stories have mythic stature as ways to perceive the world and our place in it; they also offer syntheses of many kinds of knowledge—sensuous, medical, intuitive, intellectual, tribal, biological, emotional, personal, social, and linguistic—that help us interpret our existence.

A Match to the Heart is a positive story, not simply because she gets well, but because she affirms the realities she lives in and rediscovers various wonders of nature and her body, as well as relationships between humans and between humans and nature, from small marine creatures to her faithful dogs. She writes, "It is no wonder we neglect the natural world outside ourselves when we do not have the interest to know the one within."

My review of hearts in literature well underway, I'm anxious to hear what stories Kay uses to buoy her up, in particular, from the world of rodeos.

RIDING THE WILD ANIMAL OF THE HEART; OR, BUSTING BRONCOS AND THE NASTY PILL TRAY

December 2, and the days are getting shorter and shorter. The worst wintry blasts from Canada have not yet arrived in Missoula, although it seems plenty cold to this Floridian. I'm glad I'm not in the place called, ironically, Wisdom, which—even though it's south of here—is one of the coldest spots in Montana, owing to its huge bowl shape that holds frigid air; it can go for days below zero degrees.

I've called Kay to have lunch one more time before I fly home to Florida. We've agreed to meet in a café downtown, and I'm standing in front of it, cocooned in my large winter coat, scarf, hat, and gloves, but shivering nonetheless. I see Montanan Kay coming down the street; she's wearing a light jacket not even buttoned. She's swinging her purse and whistling. Since she's not wearing a hat, her long black hair carries freely behind her.

We've barely sat down inside and she's complaining about the ESPN2 coverage of the National Finals Rodeo.

"They just don't show enough!" she says about the two and a half hours offered. "I mean, this is the Olympics of rodeos. They should show every minute of every event!"

I ask her what attracts her to rodeos.

"Well, they're inspiring. They lift me up. When I got my diagnosis, I was a basket case. I went home and got in a bad way, feeling sorry for myself. *I'm going to eat some worms,* you know? I was lying in bed, pretty well crushed, using my remote to flip through channels on the television, and I came across a rodeo event. I started watching and kept watching. It was a complete accident, or should I say an instance of grace? Rodeo—a metaphor for life. Whether it's the timed events or the rough stock . . ."

"Rough stock?"

"Oh, sorry. Rough stock includes bareback, saddle bronc, and bull riding. The timed events are steer racing, calf roping, team roping, and barrel racing. And then there's your all-around."

"Right. Inspiring?"

"These are people taking chances with large animals—right in front of a crowd right there, not to mention the television audience. They've got drive, they've got resolve, they're taking risks. I respect that. I take risks with my heart every day and every night, not because I choose to, but because I must. I'll never ride a bull or even a saddlebred horse—I'm a townie, but I identify with the rodeo competitors because they're out there, *doing it.* And doing it every day . . . like I do. Maybe my heart's the wild animal that I have to ride."

Our sandwiches arrive. I pick mine up and start to eat. Kay's sits there on her plate as she continues. "Most rodeo folks don't make any money, but they're risking life and limb. Especially the Senior Rodeo folks . . . can you imagine? They may be old, but they're up there on a wild beast, day after day, year after year. They get dumped in the dirt . . . sore . . . injured. But they get back up and ride again. I mean the Little Britches kids may not know any better, or their parents push them into it. But the older people. . . ."

She drinks from her iced tea. Iced tea! For all I know, it's snowing outside.

"And another thing: most of these folks are from small places. Just regular country people who care about what they do. It takes real gumption."

"Unlikely heroes, even country bumpkins, go way back," I say. Perceval (or Parsifal), Robin Hood, even Jesus Christ come to mind.

"Oh, it's great. I've seen some of the guys at little, dinky rodeos here in Montana who are now on national television. Some of them are in Las Vegas right now at the Nationals." She picks up her sandwich.

"How are you feeling?"

"This is a good day. I love good days. Bad days, I don't laugh at all, and it's either my illness or, more likely, the drugs getting out of balance. I'm taking several, you know, and my problem, besides being sick, is finding the right adjectives to tell the doctor. If I knew more of the exact terms and what was out of whack, that might save me some trips to the emergency room—especially at night and on weekends.

"Fortunately, my co-workers are great. If I get a little cranky, they say, 'Kay, did you take *all* of your meds this morning?' I don't often miss, but sometimes

I have them all out on the counter and sail right by them, you know, thinking of something else. Sometimes I'll be dragging at work and they'll say, 'Go home.' Which I do. I go home, take the meds, go to sleep immediately. But it can take a couple of days to get balanced again. Or you just miss something when you make up the tray."

"Is that one of the plastic things with the little boxes for each day?"

"Yeah, all the days of the week, each with its little door. That way you know you've taken Tuesday's for sure and don't skip or double up. On the one hand, it's a big help. On the other, it's big pain in the ass. All those little doors, four for each day. Sometimes I think of that nasty plastic thing as a prison. My ball and chain." She pauses.

"On the other hand . . . let's be frank. If I don't take my meds, I can be dead in six months. Clear?"

"Very clear."

"Yeah, when Dr. Knapp said that he really got my attention. Even allowing for some exaggeration to help motivate me, I know from my own body that I would be going downhill fast without my drugs. And I know from the echo numbers . . . I told you about those, right?"

"Yes."

We're silent for a moment.

"And then there are just wacky things. Winters in Montana mean that you have to always have three days' extra supply in case of a bad snowstorm. Sometimes I have to cover the office in the evening. That means I have to remember to bring my dinnertime meds to the office on that day, or my dosages are three hours late, which can mess me up.

"You know, a chore like that—which you don't even like to do. I mean, jeez, there are days when I don't want to see another pill, when I want to throw the tray on the floor and stomp on it, jump up and down on it. But you do it fifty-two weeks a year, year after year; it's so routine but still not entirely comfortable that it's easy to let your mind wander and just make a mistake, leave one out, or put in one when it should be two. Or you run out of meds and say, 'Oh, I'll have a new bottle by that day.' And then that doesn't happen, maybe in part because you accidentally-on-purpose don't want to go by the pharmacy, and you wait until it's closed. It's hard to explain to anyone who hasn't had to do the routine year after year."

"Yeah, I don't have anything like that in my experience. The closest would be brushing my teeth."

"Not even close. I take seven medications a day at three different times. Every day. Sure, I brush my teeth too, but it doesn't really matter when or if you miss a brushing.

"Now this potassium, for example. I hate to admit it, but it has really helped. It took a month to find the right level. If I miss a dose, my energy goes down the drain, and I get really moody. Yell at people, even at work. And they'll say, 'Kay, did you take your potassium?' They're great.

"And of course the doctor. You've got to have faith in your doctor. He—or she—is a source of support, and companionship and, most of all, hope. I don't know if they teach that in med school, but they should. The smart ones learn it or know it by instinct."

Kay drinks her iced tea.

"I think hope is the strongest thing I have going for me." She pauses. "I believe in fate, too. I have to believe that my illness happened to me for a reason. Somehow it's got to help others."

She's still holding her glass in the air. "That's another thing. I had to give up drinking—bad for my heart, they say, and certainly doesn't go with all the drugs I'm taking. And I've got to tell you, I really enjoyed a good glass of wine. People I used to drink with—socially, you know—now ask me, 'Does it bother you for us to have wine while you don't?' And I say, 'Well, I'm sure the wine would be nice, but, my sparkling grape juice means I'm staying healthy, and that's what means the most to me.' My biggest vice now is caffeine, but only up to 7 P.M. After that it's decaf."

"Did the doc tell you all this?"

"Heavens, no. You've got to become your own coach, manager, whatever. I've had to make up my own rules—beyond the doctor's. So, if I'm getting a cold, it's bed rest immediately, instead of dragging around. I get over it faster. It's a matter of my own experience. Docs just don't have the full picture, for one thing, and everyone's different anyway. Now me, I'm an extrovert: I need people. My friends and I always went to the gym together. We still do, but I can't do weights or keep the same pace they do. So we coordinate with my yoga schedule. We used to drink together but that's limited now, so we do other things, like beading, embroidery, or rodeo. We're on e-mail together. We talk on the phone. My friends prop me up when I'm down."

We're finishing up our sandwiches.

"These pills—if I can come back to them. . . . You know, this is an antidrug culture. If I'm out for a meal and have to take them, people stare at me, my tray, the whole deal. I used to take them into the bathroom, but I got stared at in there even worse, like I was doing dope, so I just take them in full view in the restaurant. If people want to stare, that's their problem. I'm trying to stay healthy. I have to accept my way of life as what I choose to do.

"Chronic illness is really tough. You've got it forever. It can wear you down, wear you out, or you can deal with it. I'm doing fine right now. I'm *living*. I'm looking for new challenges, new interests. I may get sicker—I understand that. I may react differently to the drugs. I may need a heart transplant. I may—I will, like all of us—die. It's just that I know what's most likely to end my life, and people without a chronic disease have no idea. In a sense, they're not oriented to one of the major facts of life. And while I wouldn't ever have chosen to have this disease, in a way I'm glad for what it has taught me."

"And what's that?"

"I'm a day-to-day athlete, someone training in illness. I have to know my own physical being—something pretty rare in America, except for athletes. If I get a nosebleed, that means I skip yoga for a day. And I have to know my mental status, so I don't get depressed. If I'm feeling sad, I know who to call. I know I need light. Up here, winters are long and dark. Furthermore, we have a lot of cloud cover here in the valley. Some folks get the SAD, seasonal affective disorder. I think I told you I'm borderline. So I got them to put in full-spectrum lights at work over my desk. I have a desk by the window. I eat my lunch outside as often as possible. Light and potassium are somehow linked, but the mechanism is not fully understood. Sleep is good; exercise is good. For me it's a pyramid, and I need every brick from the bottom up. Science will have to catch up to what some people already know through experience. I know what strategies work for me. Last winter, I had no colds, no depressive episodes, no cabin fever. A lot of regular healthy people can't claim that!" She laughs. I think of physician-poet John Stone's formulation: "Health is whatever works and for as long."

She continues, "Technical knowledge is great for people who can do it and understand it. I'm fairly sharp on various topics, but I've looked up stuff on the Internet about hearts and drugs—hard-core medical information—and I can't understand the first thing about it. That's where a good doctor is worth his weight in gold . . . to select the right stuff for each patient and to explain it in terms of that patient's world."

The waitress brings our check.

"It's a paradox. My health is poor, but I feel really good most of the time. Some days I can conquer the world. Some days I have to stay up to 2 A.M. to watch the rodeos. It's a matter of priority and strategy."

I'm impressed and tell her so.

"Yeah, well, I have friends who say they're so proud of me, blah, blah, blah, tell me I have courage, etc. I don't know whether it's courage, stubbornness, or dumb luck. I just call it living my life. Those rodeo guys fall off the horse and get back on. They do that day after day, beating the crap out of their bodies and coming back for more. If they can do it, I can too. I can take all my pills—for as long as I need to."

We part, and I walk back to the hospital. It seems to me that Kay's story, in the broadest sense, is a form of the basic quest myth. She's entered a world of obstacles, against which she's devised various strategies for action and for maintaining her resolve. Her beloved rodeo competitors are guiding lights, heroes in a parallel world of adventure and obstacles. I like the bestiality of the adversaries, the earthiness of the place, and the generally circular (or oval) form of the arena, a place that focuses yet turns about itself, a wheel of fortune, so to speak. She has, as well, a narrative of her illness, a story that tells about her past, her present, and what might exist in her future. Although she is by nature quiet and modest, I see her as the heroine of her own story.

QUALITIES OF TIME, QUALITIES OF MIND (SECOND ESSAY)

Modern medicine has been traditionally divided into two wings—surgical and medical, the latter referring to the use of pharmaceuticals, or drugs. Michael had a surgical solution to his heart dilemma, a problem which came into his life within a short time span and which had a correspondingly short treatment time. Furthermore, his faulty valve had a spatial dilemma that could be well shown by X-rays and sonograms, allowing the diagnosis to be made relatively quickly. Kay, on the other hand, is a medical cardiac patient who works with an internist, not a surgeon. No scalpel can enter her heart and repair the damage; no balloon can adjust her arteries. Her chronic heart disease and diagnosis emerged slowly; her medicines took a year to balance, and still must be checked. Further—as she counts her pills, assesses her activities and energies every day, and reports to her doctor—she is a student of her own condition, co-writing, so to speak, the narrative of her treatment. No one can show her the virus that weakened her heart muscles; her heart's illness was mysterious, absurd, and the limitations of her heart are chronic, continuous, and—unless a miracle or a medical breakthrough occurs—companions for the rest of her life. Doctors attributed Michael's valve deformation to an embryological error, a defined event, a clear story of origin that explains the dilemma. Kay has no similarly satisfying explanation. Her illness possibly originated with a virus, not a well-defined event. In a culture that likes explanations and certainty, such mysterious origins can be troubling, even though she has shaped a general story that accounts for her heart failure and that sketches possible futures.

As for the long run, Michael appears to be at no more risk than anyone else. His future time and its quality is comparable to other twenty-eight-year-old males. Time for Kay has a different quality. Despite all her faithfulness to regimen and her self-imposed strategies, her heart may get worse. She sees the possibility of a heart transplant but knows an AB positive heart is hard to find. Some three thousand people need new hearts in America at this writing; some of them wait a year or more. Many die while waiting. While all of us are mortal, Kay has a clearer sense of a story that may control the end of her life. The origin of her illness is lost in time, but her well-defined illness may cause the end of her life. (Of course, her life may end sooner for other reasons—as any of our lives may.)

The root of the word "medicine" is *medicus,* Latin for doctor, telling us that this role has existed in society for at least two millennia, even if theories and techniques have changed greatly. The dictionary gives other concepts in the related words, "measure," "reflect," even "meditate," all suggesting qualitative ways the mind may work. But not only does Dr. Knapp weigh and balance

Kay's medications, patient Kay weighs and balances her energy expenditures, her stress, her exposure to sunlight. She sees herself as one of her caregivers, an athlete at the center of her very own rodeo corral. She is the heroine of a night-sea journey, like Jonah who sank in the sea, dwelt in the whale, but popped back up, or Melville's Ishmael, saved from the sea by Queequeg's coffin.

How do we live with hearts, sick or well? Kay takes her meds, gets rest, and measures out her energy. One of Kay's practices is yoga, an ancient tradition whose name relates to our modern word "yoke." The yoking or joining sought is between Atman and Brahman, or self and the encompassing All, or the individual person and the godhead. Americans often practice it in more secular terms, yoking mind and body, yoking self and a more general quality, such as enlightenment or peace. In Hindu tradition the energies of the body are organized by seven chakras that line up along the spine. The center one is the heart chakra (anahata), a transition between the three lower chakras (anus, genitals, belly) and the three upper (throat, third eye, crown). Thus it participates in the lower, more animal aspects of humans and also in the upper, more cerebral and spiritual aspects. There is considerable esoteric lore attached to this chakra, typically revolving around love, devotion, and compassion. There is even a report of a Swami Rama intentionally stopping (and restarting) his heart by using yoga in an experiment at the Menninger Foundation in 1971. I imagine western medicine will learn more of links between the heart and the brain, but Kay has already developed her own, based on her awareness of her own mind and body. While the root of the word "patient" means "one who suffers," our modern sense of "one who undergoes medical treatment" and "one who is tolerant or calm" also applies to resilient Kay.

In another sense of the word "yoke," the connection of a heart patient and a loving, devoted, compassionate doctor would be ideal, as in the case of Gretel Ehrlich and Dr. Braniff. In a dynamic doctor-patient relationship—and especially with a chronic illness—knowledge of health and illness flows back and forth between doctor and patient in this creative, dynamic yoke. Moderns are so attuned to motor vehicles that it is hard to remember most of the history of agriculture depended upon the yoke, a means of hitching an animal to a plow, a wagon, a sled. To what powers, ideas, faiths do each of us yoke ourselves?

One night I watch bull riding on television, in honor of Kay. The word "rodeo" originally meant the pen or the corral for cattle; now it means the competition itself of cowboy skills within that space; the word comes from the Spanish "rota," or wheel, a roundness that reminds me of the organic heart. The arena is generally a dirt area surrounded by walls and bleachers for the spectators. An analogue to the larger world, the space is animated by people and animals;

here we have well-defined forces, as in football games, racetracks, boxing rings, or the gladiatorial Colosseum of ancient Rome. While the conflict is external to us, as spectators we participate emotionally as we watch a dramatic and immediate ritual of strength and technique, humans vs. large beasts, with very real danger to both. It's been some thirty years since I attended an actual rodeo (which was in rural Missouri), and I'm surprised how vivid, how close-up the long lenses of television cameras can now make the event.

TV gives me startling views of slender, athletic men on top of monstrous bulls, fourteen hundred pounds or more of muscle tensed and waiting for the gate to swing open. With a tight flank strap around their hindquarters and the pricks of the cowboys' spurs, the bulls erupt into explosive bucks and turns, often pitching the cowboys off. The rider hangs with one hand to his rope around the bull's chest, gaining points for form and, of course, for the length of his ride. He tries to stay on for eight seconds—which often doesn't happen. If he "makes the whistle," he jumps off as best he can and seeks the safety of the rodeo clowns rushing in to distract the bull. If the cowboy is *thrown* off, he is especially glad to see the rodeo clowns, because he has little control over his fall to the ground, where the bull may step on him or even gore him. I'm amazed that humans would choose to ride bulls, voluntarily risking injury; indeed it's the most injury-prone event of the rodeo. One rider reports that getting hit by a bull is like being hit by a truck traveling at twenty miles per hour. Kay sees the life of these cowboys as analogous to her struggles with her heart and draws inspiration from them. I'd like to stretch her comparison further and consider the rodeo clown's role as analogous to a doctor's.

Like circus clowns, rodeo clowns wear goofy outfits, with funny hats and dangling scarves; they wear makeup to exaggerate their eyes and mouths. They often have wild stripes or polka dots in their clothing, but they do not wear the extra-large shoes of the circus clown because they need to be nimble in the corral. While they may look oafish, they are in fact athletes who deal directly with danger: an alternate name for them is, in fact, "bullfighter." As a rider goes down, they must protect him from the bull; they run toward the bull and distract it, waving their arms and yelling. Their clownish clothes mark them as different from the competing cowboys in regular western garb of jeans, hat, and a number pinned on their backs, much as a doctor's lab coat, scrubs, or stethoscope defines his or her role. When a rodeo clown gets older, when he—and it almost always is a man—has had enough injuries (spine, knee, ribs, and, especially, concussions), he often becomes a barrel man, luring the bull away from the fallen rider and climbing into a custom-made barrel that no animal can crush. Sometimes the barrel man provides comedy acts between events or works a microphone—a crowd pleaser.

Doctors intervene in our lives when the bull throws us. They take away (distract) the illness by whatever means they can. Doctors have the training and experience that accustoms them to illness and injury. They have seen mangled limbs. They have seen patients die. When we go to their offices, we have faith that they know the best and worst outcomes possible and that they are able to face these with us and give us comfort and hope. Kay said that faith in her doctor was central to her perspective on her disease.

And clownishness? Clowns make us laugh, reawakening childish glee in us, a deep resource for being truly human. A good doctor helps us technically, of course, but a great doctor puts us at ease and relates as person to person, not as strong to weak, nor as well to sick. A great doctor knows when humor will help, so that he and the patient can join in laughing, can team up against any bull. (Patch Adams and his Gesundheit Institute come to mind, but less famous docs—including any who treat me—can always win my heart with good humor.) The dictionary tells me that the words "clown" and "clod" are related, suggesting a rustic peasant, the unlikely hero, a man of the soil—hence a boorish fellow, one without the niceties of city folk. The rodeo clown works in the churned up soil of the rodeo, truly a man of the earth. He pretends to be silly, but his work partakes of life and death, the rider's and his own. The words "human" and "humus" are related, but we have largely divorced ourselves from the soil, living in cities, traveling in cars, fearing any *dirt* in our living spaces. With Dr. Grant we got closer to the *prima materia* of working hearts, the neurotransmitters and ions that made the individual muscle cells contract. Some of these sound so simple—sodium, calcium, potassium—common elements that work with the carbon, oxygen, nitrogen, and hydrogen that make up 96 percent of us and a lot of the rest of nature, even the stars. And yet, reaching this elemental level does not disclose any absolute essence of the heart, only another level of its wonderful efficiency and complexity.

Doctors who work with children often wear ties with cartoon animals for the distraction and amusement of their patients. (They used to attach a little furry animal to their stethoscopes for the same purpose until these were judged to be germ-transfer stations.) Such simple techniques—clownish gestures—can do wonders by bringing positive qualities such as joy, playfulness, even freedom (all heart values) into doctor-patient encounters that are stressful for children and parents. Many years ago, while traveling in Ireland, my wife and I were awakened by terrible coughs coming from our daughter; we could hear them through a hotel wall. Alarmed, we asked the night clerk to call for a doctor, who came in the middle of the night, friendly and kind. Upon greeting our daughter, he asked to listen to her teddy bear's heart. When she assented, he placed the end of his stethoscope on the bear's chest and listened earnestly.

Then he asked if he could listen to her heart, and she pulled up her pajama top with lightning speed. After examining his cooperative patient, he said the cough was not dangerous. And then he, the night clerk, and I had a cup of tea in the hotel's parlor. In a brief time, in the middle of an Irish night, because of the kindness of a doctor and a night clerk, my mind shifted from anxiety and fear to calmness and gratitude.

I look over my notes for Michael and Kay. A Cartesian mania seizes me, and I start to sketch out a comparative grid:

	What Is the Heart? Two Views	
Person/Patient	Michael	Kay
Heart as ailment	Hemodynamic organ Incompetent valve	Biochemical wonder Viral cardiomyopathy
Branch of medicine	Cardiac surgery	Cardiology (internal medicine)
Medical intervention	Ross procedure (surgery)	Pharmaceuticals
Patient's concept(s) of the heart	Basis for life, athletics	A wild animal to ride, to manage
Patient strategies	Rehab, family, friends, words	Friends, yoga, rodeos, counseling
Humanistic perspective	Words	Stories
Outcome aim	Healthy valves	Adequate ejection fraction
Major metaphor	Gift	Miracle (see below)

As a comparativist, I'm pleased with this grid. It's clear, orderly, and wonder-fully rectilinear. At the same time, I'm uneasy with its Cartesian rectitude. The old Malvina Reynolds song about "little boxes" starts up in my mind, and I sense that my structure is unheartlike in form and spirit, although perhaps revealing in its content. Indeed it looks a lot like the "napkin schematic" we saw earlier, everything linear and separated by lines—part of the story, but not suggestive enough.

What is the problem here? Information is put into squares, little rooms, or chambers. We speak of *chambers of the heart,* a phrase that gives authority and grandeur. What other chambers do we know? The chambers of a judge, the chambers of a legislature. My lady's chambers. Or power, as in chambers of a gun. A chamberlain is an important person. A chambermaid works in a rich person's house. Chamber music is definitely upscale. We don't say "rooms of the heart," which is about as accurate, perhaps because rooms can be rented,

Alcove Model: Two Perspectives on the Heart

a. Person
b. A biological definition of heart
c. Diagnosed illness(es)

d. Branch of treating medicine
e. Medical intervention(s)
f. Patient concept(s) of heart
g. Patient support strategies

h. Humanistic perspective
i. Outcome aim
j. Exemplary metaphor

a. **Michael**
b. Hemodynamic organ
c. Incompetent valve
d. Cardiac surgery
e. Ross procedure
f. Basis for life, athletics
g. Rehab, family, friends, words
h. Words, naming of parts
i. Healthy valves
j. Gift

OUR
HUMAN
HEART

a. **Kay**
b. Biochemical wonder
c. Viral cardiomyopathy
d. Cardiology, internal medicine
e. Pharmaceuticals
f. A wild animal to ride, to manage
g. Friends, yoga, rodeos, counseling
h. Stories
i. Adequate ejection fraction
j. Miracle

Alcove Model showing two perspectives of the heart. The curved lines here suggest that each alcove is a set of perspectives on the heart, perceiving it and defining it in a particular way.

generic spaces of no intrinsic value. But at the anatomy lab or the butcher's shop we find that the chambers of the heart are *not* cubic in form, nor do they hold themselves open waiting for blood to come in. They have curved walls, with stabilizing cords through them. At death, they collapse, like the deer heart I examined earlier. I'm considering organic shapes now, not the industrial or architectural right angles that pervade modern mass society. Chakras are round, rodeos are oval or round, the earth is round.

Besides, the meanings I'm finding in Michael and Kay clearly have overlap; they are not in discrete boxes, chambers, or rooms. I redraw my comparison, using the concept of *alcove,* a niche, or vault, an arched opening in a larger room of the heart as a whole. ("Vault" relates to roundness, as in the vault of the skull; its Latin root is *volvere,* "to roll.") These two alcoves—one for Michael, one for Kay—provide two perspectives on the heart. In each one the scientific and the humanistic overlap. In Michael, we saw that words and numbers, terms and graphs were subsets of a larger set of metaphors, ways of coming to terms with the heart. In Kay, we saw that stories were linear narratives that a doctor or a patient could construct to make sense of a patient's case.

And what could be a central metaphor for the heart, given all we've seen in Kay's section? I remember Dr. Grant's use of the word "miraculous" to describe the swift and continuous neurohumoral changes in cardiac muscle, as well as the intricate mind-heart, mind-vasculature connections at work, minute by minute, in our bodies. So, I pick the word "miracle." A miracle, the dictionary tells me, is something to be wondered at or admired—a cognate word. The miracle can be religious, as in Jesus's acts, or secular, as in a glorious sunset, a narrow escape from harm, or a birth. The operative concept concerning hearts, I think, lies in the perceiver: we can consider the heart as a miracle only if we reflect on what it does, how it works, how it originated, how very long it may last. Like the proverbial tree falling in the forest, its miraculous sound (and I mean beyond heartbeats) is perceived only if there is a perceiver, but unlike that tree, it beats day and night whether or not we perceive it. And perceivers? Any of us, of course, but I think especially of clowns or persons who delight in clowns, persons who feel joy, who affirm and celebrate what they perceive.

Steve's Angina Pectoris and
Change of Stories

Among the People

The heart ailments of Michael and Kay came upon them regardless of their behavior, activities, or health risks. Michael's faulty valve came—perhaps—from an embryological oddity; Kay's pericarditis/endocarditis came—perhaps—from an immune system weakness. With Steve, whose cardiac illness illustrates this section, we turn to a wider approach to health and illness, epidemiology, which studies classes of diseases amongst an entire population. One cause of disease can be behavioral, how we live day to day and under what stresses. Epidemiology studies health behaviors, health risks, and the incidence of disease within groups of people—nations, tribes, towns, meat-eaters, smokers, inhabitants around a Love Canal. The basis of the word is, of course, "epidemic," but even further we have the Greek roots, *epi* and *demos,* or "among the people." When I observed at the Centers for Disease Control and Prevention (CDC) in Atlanta, Georgia, I listened to an administrator for the Epidemic Intelligence Services talk on his speaker phone with teams far flung to points all over the globe. As he spoke with them, he pointed out to me the corresponding flags pinned on a large world map on the wall. His colleagues afield were Atlanta-based epidemiologists who can board a plane with their gear on twenty-four-hours' notice to analyze a poisoning at a restaurant or track down a mysterious illness, such as a hanta virus in the American southwest. Such trips are perhaps the most dramatic work of epidemiologists. But epidemiological studies, which can rely heavily on statistical analysis, are also important for understanding larger issues, such as nutrition, water and air quality, health habits, and more—issues that are basic to the health of all our citizens. In the last thirty years, the CDC has helped to figure out Legionnaire's disease, AIDS, toxic shock syndrome, and links between street drugs and hepatitis.

The CDC also works on environmental health, as well as health promotion and education. Applied epidemiology, so to speak, is the basis for such public health services as sanitation, health screenings, inoculations, well baby visits, and even routine physicals. Public health is interested not only in fighting disease but in promoting healthy lives of long length and good quality. From ancient times, medicine has dealt with illness and injury, but the nineteenth-century triumphs in nutrition, germ theory, and antisepsis, and the twentieth-century advances in drugs (such as antibiotics and anesthesia), vitamins, genetics, and, again, epidemiology, have dramatically reduced the incidences of communicable diseases and many injuries (think of advances in workplace safety) in the so-called developed countries. Without cholera, typhoid, and tuberculosis, we now live long enough to die of degenerative diseases of old age—heart disease, cancer, and neurological diseases such as Parkinson's. But are there environmental factors for cancer? Cluster outbreaks suggest such links, as shown in the movie *Erin Brockovich*. Clearly this will be a growing field of epidemiological study as we find our environments increasingly influenced by chemicals, increasingly crowded, and increasingly influenced by world travel. Further understanding of preventing heart disease and cancers may benefit us all.

There are also social and psychological factors to health: the behaviors prevalent within a culture. With lifestyles that are urban, fast-paced, competitive, and performance-oriented, we find pervasive stress. These factors have been studied and are now often a part of a doctor's conversation with an adult patient during a routine physical, in which, ideally, a doctor will discuss family history, current health practices and risks (including diet, exercise, alcohol and tobacco usage), and stressors. Sometimes these are ignored, although journalistic accounts of them are widely available. Sometimes it's an event of cardiac illness that scares a woman or man into changing behaviors in order to lessen the risk of future cardiac trouble.

In front of the red-brick buildings of the CDC, there's a bust of Hygeia, the ancient Greek goddess of health. Institutional medicine has largely followed Apollo, the healer of illness, the active archetype for wielding the scalpel or prescribing drugs in response to trauma and illness. But Hygeia is now having her day as well. Not only is she cost effective, but our mothers have kept her alive by teaching us personal hygiene, feeding us well, and reminding us to dress right for the weather. Some fifty years later I can remember my mother telling me about Calvin Coolidge's son, who died from a foot infection because he didn't change his socks!

We have looked at explicit, conscious stories in Kay's section, stories constructed by authors, doctors, and patients. In Steve's section, we will look at implicit or unconscious stories, narratives that guide our behavior even though we are unaware of them. Some of these are not healthy. To help heal his heart, Steve needed to uncover such stories and replace them.

A Strangling of the Chest

"I was lifting a piano—which I probably shouldn't have been doing in any case—but there I was, and suddenly I felt incredible pain." Steve Oreskovich, an Episcopal priest, is talking with me in his study at the church. When I heard he had heart trouble, I asked to interview him. His pain, I learned, was angina pectoris—literally, "a strangling of the chest."

"It was just crushing and left me gasping, totally weak. I also had asthma, so I had ignored all previous hints, such as tiredness, trouble breathing, and so on; I just blamed my asthma. Easy, huh? Besides, I was in great shape, at least by some measures; I was capable of fourteen-mile-a-day hikes, that sort of thing. I had a terrible diet, though—mostly cheese pizza—and I didn't handle stress well at all. Looking back, it's obvious: the bishop had just come to visit my church. I was anxious, worried. I could lose my job—a job I liked a lot."

Steve's church, Holy Spirit Episcopal, is in a Missoula neighborhood of old, large houses. It's a stone church with adjoining buildings all shaped in a U around a green lawn. The roofs, which have sharp pitches to dump off snow, have recently been redone in costly slate with copper trim, which still shines brightly before weathering to a dull green. Steve's office was the living room of the manse for earlier rectors. At fifty-one, he's a vibrant man with black hair and a black beard, both touched by gray. He gestures as he talks.

"So I went to the doctor, who did an EKG. He immediately said, 'Go home and pick up your shaving kit. We're going to the hospital.' OK, so we went. An angiogram showed partial blockage in my coronary vessels, so I had angioplasty to open them up." For angioplasty, a doctor snakes a catheter up from a puncture in the groin, through blood vessels, to the heart; guided by X-rays, he inserts the end of the catheter into constricted areas of the coronary artery and inflates a balloon to compress the plaque and open up the lumen—the interior space of the artery. He can also introduce a stent, a tubular wire cage that supports the artery from within. When I watched these procedures in Chapel Hill, they appeared to be some kind of magic. The interventional radiologist marked the problem areas on the X-ray with his red marker then went after them with his catheter. Fifteen minutes later, he was done.

Steve continues. "My doc said that I'd be dead in five years without modern technology. And so I soldiered on ... emotions were to come later. I was basically *on hold* for six months, living in fear, really, and slowly wondering what life meant, and what did my own fragility mean?

"I had been a chaplain's assistant in the Army, where I dealt with Vietnam vets, so I had some idea of how to take care of other people. I just didn't seem to know how to take care of myself. In sum, I went into a six-month depression.

I could understand that my body needed rest, but I had a more difficult time understanding that my mind—or is it my soul?—also needed rest. R and R. Revitalization . . . re-creation, in the literal sense. It's what all the men's groups have been about: coming to terms with lack of control in a society that prizes control, especially by men. Coming to terms with insecurity in a society that assumes we are all secure, and, of course, the famous one—coming to terms with emotions. In this culture men are all supposed to be John Wayne characters. *It's only a flesh wound. Shake it off. Play hurt. Win one for the Gipper.*" Shaking our heads from side to side, Steve and I laugh the quiet sardonic laugh of men who have lived this crap, who have acted out these pathetic stories of hyper-responsibility and perfection, but also it's a celebrative chuckle of men who have also tried to refashion their lives. I have been in men's groups where I and others complained loudly about the pressures we felt at work, at home—everywhere. I too have lived the First-Child, Protestant-Work-Ethic, Type-A-Behavior Pattern: *Let's do everything, be perfect, and do it all very fast!* But Steve has been there on the cold steel table for his angioplasty, and I have not.

"They put about a five-pound bag of sand on my crotch to encourage the wound to clot and close up," Steve continues. "And there I am, looking at the ceiling, feeling blood dripping down my leg. And some guys get these things like they get haircuts. I know one man who's had five of them.

"I was living the whole tight thing . . . all shielded by various mental and physical postures . . . a hard-shell of defense. Do good! Be perfect!" Steve and I are sitting in comfortable chairs that are at a ninety-degree angle. We can look at each other or not, as we choose. Between us in the corner is a low table with a lamp and a box of tissues. I realize this is where Steve counsels some of his parishioners. I imagine he's very good at it . . . the wounded healer. The guy who has *been there.*

"I should have seen it coming all along. My dad died of a heart attack when he was forty-two . My cholesterol was up to 316. I was overweight. What a fine collection of risk factors! So I had no excuses for getting sick. And I got treated and started on the drugs." Steve pauses.

"But then I realized I didn't understand what life meant . . . and me a minister, right? Here I was forty years old and suddenly ground down. I began to entertain fantasies . . . I'd quit my job and write or paint. I'd enter the computer world. I'd run away. Suddenly I was *manic,* making up wild stories . . . as opposed to some men I counsel with, who are basically locked in, stifled. Oh, we can dig the rut so deep." He saws the air with the side of his hand.

"My wife, Brenda, was great all through this, though. Not that it was always easy. We had a lot of trouble at first and went to a marital counselor. What an irony—I mean, I *do* marital counseling routinely for other folks, but this was a different matter, something I couldn't magically solve. Brenda kept saying she just wanted things back to normal. And I was sick . . . I couldn't make decisions . . . I felt impotent, totally beat. In counseling I said we were a couple of punch-drunk fighters. Brenda loved that; we finally had some language for things we were keeping hidden, from each other, from ourselves. We were both afraid, but putting up good fronts for each other. Shields, you know? We were both angry and repressing that. She hated my disease and could finally say so. Just putting language to all these things got us halfway to healing. It clarified everything and gave us some solid footing."

Solid footing. What do Americans assume is solid? A house? A career? A title? Money? The language of Steve's counseling gave some definition to feelings—another kind of solidity—that were below the surface. At the same time, Steve was also making up wild stories, new scenarios for his life. Some of the old stories that drove him had not been clear to him, tacit or implicit stories that the angina helped bring to consciousness, the old stories of *the little engine that could,* Horatio Alger, any boy can be president, and even poor old John Henry, swinging his hammer to beat the steam drill until he died. *Strive, be number one, be perfect, take control!* And, of course, build up social position and wealth.

Solid footing. As I walk back to the hospital, I think about my shoes on the sidewalk, and the earth underneath, largely a jumble of rocks and soil brought down to this valley by glaciers from Canada. I also think of Antaeus, the giant of classical antiquity who derived strength from his mother, Gaea, the earth. Hercules could strangle him only by lifting him from the earth, his source. I've read commentary that the moderns—in their cars, their buildings, their cities—have lost touch with the earth and the strength it might offer. Many have gone "back to the land," like Steve, as we shall see.

Mrs. Sanders Dies in the ER

If Steve's illness had been left untreated, it most likely would have led to a heart attack. Such an event might have been fatal, since a person suffering a heart attack can die on the spot, especially if he or she has had an attack before. While we commonly think of heart attack victims as being men, women suffer them too; cardiologists commonly say that they have them "ten years later," after they have passed menopause and they lose hormonal protection. Because women's symptoms tend to be more diffuse and harder for doctors (and the women themselves) to recognize, there are sometimes delays in treatment. As with trauma patients, there's a Golden Hour, the sixty minutes during which medical treatment can make a tremendous difference. Accordingly, a patient presenting with chest pain will be designated "ROMI," meaning "rule out myocardial infarction," in order to guard against a worst case of a heart attack in progress. Even if a woman arrives at a hospital or clinic shortly after becoming ill, however, the correct diagnosis may take longer than for men, thus further delaying medical intervention. Indeed, some 250,000 American women die of heart attacks each year—roughly four times the mortality of breast cancer. And yet women fear breast cancer more and often ignore factors that could save them from heart disease. Men don't do any better, fearing cancer but choosing to lead stress-filled lives. While stress was a factor in Steve's illness, stress is not always a cause or even an intensifier for cardiac illness. In the following case, the patient history of stress or any other risks was not known, because it was an emergency.

It's Wednesday afternoon, my usual time to volunteer in the Emergency Room/Trauma Center of Bayfront Medical Center. A six-hundred-bed hospital in downtown St. Petersburg, we get plenty of business. Ambulances roll up to our doors with regularity, and three medically equipped helicopters land on our roof with patients from up to 250 miles away. The ER has some thirty beds, including two critical care rooms, CCA and CCB. It is in CCB that two nurses—alerted by radio—await the arrival of a woman I'll call Lucia Sanders.

The radio connects us to ambulances across the county. Today Bonnie takes the call. She writes down the patient's name, the chief complaint, vital signs, and estimated time of arrival (ETA) in a log. This patient's pulse rate is 140 and her BP (blood pressure) is falling, now 105 over 65, signs that suggest she's heading into shock. (Shock, as we saw above, means that there is inadequate blood supply to the entire body. The heart is trying to get the blood around, but the BP shows it isn't happening.) Bonnie writes on a whiteboard: "#5 [the ambulance], M.I., 10 min, CCB." This note tells the paramedics where to wheel the patient when they come through the sliding glass doors. She also alerts Jeff, the charge nurse for this shift, of the imminent arrival of "a woman with a possible M.I." and the severity of the patient's condition. He agrees that CCB is the right place, an easy choice, since CCA already has an asthmatic patient. Exactly when the attack occurred is unclear; the longer ago, the worse her chances. If she has already taken aspirin to thin her blood, that would be in her favor. Mrs. Sanders, seventy-five years old, is coming from her apartment building, where a neighbor called 911.

Upon arriving at the apartment at 3:07 P.M., paramedics found a dazed woman in much distress. She said she felt bad in the morning but thought it was just a "spell" that would pass. Now she has severe chest pain; she's sweating; she has vomited without expelling much. She complains of crushing pain in her chest, left arm, and neck. Within one of her coronary arteries, a plaque has ruptured, causing a thrombus—or clot—which blocks blood flow. Heart muscle downstream from there has been starved of oxygen and nutrients, and cells are dying. (Heart attacks often occur between 6 A.M. and noon, with a peak within the first three hours of awakening; some believe that changes in adrenocortical hormones are precipitating factors, as the body energizes from rest to action according to our intrinsic circadian rhythm.)

The two nurses don't like waiting in CCB, knowing that their still-distant patient is in danger. Furthermore, they have other patients already, and, like most people in helping professions, they want to apply their skills immediately to make a difference for the patient. They look at their watches and the clock high over the bed. They make jokes about the ambulance, that the paramedics may have stopped at a bank or paused for lunch, and they make small talk, but basically they want to get their hands on Mrs. Sanders.

The automatic doors jerk open, and the paramedics wheel in the gurney with their patient. She's a heavy woman; her white hair is matted with sweat. An oxygen mask covers her mouth and nose. She's getting an IV of dextrose and water with some epinephrine (synthetic adrenaline) to stimulate the heart. The paramedics and nurses roll the stretcher next to the bed and—on a count of three—pull her across to it. The nurses cut her clothes away, tossing them on the floor out of the way. Even though her skin is deeply pigmented—she's an African-American woman—a bluish cast is discernible, especially in her palms, nail beds, and mouth, caused by lack of oxygen. Dr. Lind, a tall woman in a white lab coat, joins the group.

"What's your name?" she asks the patient. Lucia slowly looks up at her but is too sick to answer.

"It's Lucia," a nurse says, reading from the paramedic's run sheet.

"Well, Lucia, we're going to take care of you," Dr. Lind says. "What have we got?" The paramedic and nurses give her "the bullet," a summary of the case so far. Dr. Lind orders an EKG; the machine is already there, the order expected. (Ambulances equipped for advanced life support can radio EKG results to the ER.) One nurse has been taking the four classic vital signs (pulse, blood pressure, respirations, and temperature); she places various leads for monitoring on Lucia's body. Several of us look at the screen overhead where the tracings show her pulse now at a slow 58. The automatic BP cuff is set to inflate every five minutes; it now shows 95/50. A nurse wipes Lucia's chest and puts the EKG leads onto her—six on the chest and four on the limbs—to get the electrical news of her heart. At the same time, another nurse draws blood to see what the cardiac enzymes are doing, although some of them may not show any change for hours.

Dr. Lind orders morphine for chest pain, although a small amount, since it can depress breathing and blood pressure. She orders heparin to thin the blood and TNKase to dissolve any clots, although it too has risks (such as internal bleeding). She gives her more nitroglycerine to dilate peripheral vessels and lighten the heart's load. Nonetheless, Lucia's pulse and blood pressure are still dropping; she's in bad shape.

"Epi," orders Dr. Lind, giving the amount for another shot of synthetic adrenaline.

"Any family?" Dr. Lind asks. A paramedic who has stayed to watch says no. He and I stand at the rear of the small room. The closed doors and the closed blinds on the windows guard this woman's privacy and keep other patients from observing a difficult scene. I say a silent prayer for her and for the people working on her.

"Tube her," Dr. Lind says, and a nurse inserts an endotracheal tube, which is connected to a ventilator. A respiratory therapist has arrived to oversee the settings.

Lucia's pulse continues to drop. "We're in brady land," a nurse says. (Bradycardia means the heart is beating too slowly—now at 45 bpm.) Dr. Lind calls for atropine to boost the heart rate. If this fails, a pacemaker might do the job. Everyone looks at the monitor to see if pulse increases, but we see something else.

The green line that showed electrical activity has become a chaotic scribble. "And now we've got a code," Dr. Lind says. Lucia's heart is in ventricular fibrillation, a state of disorganized contractions that can't pump blood. Persons who have felt a heart under such conditions typically say it feels like "a bag of worms," an image I find hard to forget. (Code means either the heart or breathing is not working. In hospital parlance, you can "call a code," "run a code," or—if you're a sick human being—you can simply "code," which means you're in immediate danger of dying.)

"Damn . . . v. fib," Dr. Lind says. "Zap her." A nurse applies paddles to her chest and calls "Clear!" She triggers the electrical jolt that might shock the heart out of arrhythmia and allow the regular rhythm to resume. We all watch the monitor . . . the scrawl continues. She tries two more times at higher energies. Lucia's body lurches in the bed as muscles contract from the electricity. The shocks stop the v. fib, but the heart is so damaged there is no intrinsic rhythm left to take over. Deprived of orderly cardiac output, the blood pressure plummets. The monitor's green line drifts up, drifts down, shows an occasional heartbeat, drifting sideways in an "agonal rhythm." Without oxygen, Lucia's brain is shutting down, also her kidneys, also the lining of her gut. Organ system by organ system, she is dying.

Dr. Lind has offered all that modern medicine can do. It'll take a while for the tenacious heart fibers to stop completely—these are among the last cells to die—but by medical and legal standards, this woman is now dead—except for a doctor's pronouncement. Dr. Lind looks at the clock overhead. "We'll call it at 4:12," she says, and the recording nurse writes this on the chart, the official time of death. "Someone close her eyes." Another nurse pushes the eyelids down, holds them for a moment, and then withdraws her hand. The lids start to rise again, revealing the huge black pupils of death. She pushes them down again and holds them longer. They stay down.

The respiratory therapist disconnects the vent tube, leaving the plastic endotracheal tube just protruding from the woman's mouth. He wheels his ventilator away. Crash cart and EKG machines are wheeled away. Everyone leaves the room. No one says anything. Each person turns to other patients with an air of "all in a day's work," but the truth is that doctors and nurses don't like to lose patients for any reason. Hospital norms favor saving lives at all costs, and death is generally viewed as a failure.

Driven by the IV drugs, Lucia's heart still beats occasionally, but the orderly heart-brain connection is finished, the heart-vasculature system has collapsed, and within an hour her heart will be as still as all the other tissues in her body. I look at her body, say a prayer, and wonder, when is a life acceptably over? When is death itself a form of healing?

"LIVING RIGHT COULD PUT ME OUT OF BUSINESS": STRESS PLAYSHOP

I'm having lunch with Dr. Joe Knapp; he's a cardiologist/internal medicine physician with an interest in epidemiology. I got in touch with him through Kay; he's her doctor. Midcareer, he went back to school to earn an M.P.H., a master's in public health. I've read about some of the more famous cases of diseases within a culture. One example commonly cited is Japan, which had no coronary heart disease early in this century, but which now has coronary heart disease as a number two killer, after esophageal cancer. In the United States, the Framingham Heart Study has analyzed two generations of Massachusetts families since 1948, providing much of the current information about the risk factors for coronary heart disease, such as fatty diets, smoking, lack of exercise, and stress.

We're eating lunch at a Thai restaurant, three blocks from the hospital. Joe's wearing jeans and a plaid shirt—his normal doctoring outfit. Often he carries his three-headed stethoscope, but today he's left that at the office. I gather that Joe likes this restaurant because of the healthy food. I also notice that several people wave to him: he's a regular. A small town like Missoula (pop. 75,000) has a closer downtown community than St. Petersburg (pop. 300,000). Such recognition is a social food, of sorts. If I go to a restaurant downtown in St. Petersburg, I will most likely know no one.

After we order, I ask him about the epidemiological approach to hearts.

"Heart disease is largely a disease of civilization," he says. "We have all kinds of examples of populations where heart disease was unknown until lifestyle and environmental changes came along: the car, sitting at desks, eating fatty food, loss of exercise, increase in smoking. The human body was designed to be active, to eat healthy foods, and to have rest and relaxation. And where did this design come from? Thousands and thousands of years of evolutionary development of the human body, brain, and, of course, the system that passes that along—genetics. If you count our mammalian precursors, that's millions of years. We're very well built for a lifestyle that is disappearing in the twentieth century—a mere hiccup in the larger time frame. People's lives got longer in this century because of advances in medical care, improved diets, and so on. We can treat trauma very well. Inoculations and screenings have done a wonderful job in limiting or even eliminating disease. The infectious diseases that used to kill people are pretty much out of the way. Now we live long enough to die of heart disease and cancer. Factors for cancer risk are only partially controllable . . . and there's a lot we don't know about cancer yet.

"Heart and vascular disease—our number one killer—is, on the other hand, largely controllable. We know a lot about how the heart works and what causes heart disease. Except for family history—which no one can control—we can control most of the other factors. If we did everything right, we could routinely live a long time. Leaving aside some genetic anomalies and some trauma (as from cars, for example—and we should do more about that), we could live over 100 years, and in good health. You see different estimates, but a lot of them come out at about 120 years of age. Boy, have we screwed that up!" He pauses a moment to eat.

"When I was doing work on the reservation in Arizona," Joe says, "I'd see 100 to 150 patients a day. Indians live under tough conditions, many of which are unfair, but they eat a simple diet, walk a lot, and stay active in general. Most of them have a spiritual dimension to their lives that makes some sense of the world; no matter how absurd and impoverished life is on the 'rez,' many Indians find a way to live day to day. So I'd see infectious disease, diabetes, lung problems, and routine things like that, but almost never would I see heart disease."

I mention a TV documentary I saw about the Papago Indians, a tribe on the border of Arizona and Mexico. The Arizona Papagos have more money but less physical work. They eat fast food and go to the casino to gamble. They watch TV. Many of them are fat and out of shape. They have heart disease. Their counterparts just across the border, a handful of miles away, have exactly the same genetic heritage—a constant factor in this comparison—but their diet (corn and beans) and daily activities (farming, walking, generally staying active) still follow the traditions of many centuries. They have no heart disease.

Joe mentions another case, Holland. "The Dutch had a lot of heart disease before and even during World War II. Afterwards it dropped way down. When the war stopped, suddenly they were on something close to a starvation diet. They were working hard to rebuild their country; they had something to believe in . . . they had hope. The stress of being strafed or bombed completely disappeared.

"It's so simple, it's almost laughable. I could put myself out of business with most of my patients if I could get them to manage their own health. That's really the nub: everybody makes fun of 'managed care' because they think of CEOs in office buildings making skinflinty decisions about length of stay, what procedures can be justified, and so forth—and that's a factor, sure enough. But *more important* [he gestures emphatically with his fork] and especially in the long run, corporate managed care would make out better if it became largely *preventive,* making sure doctors and patients managed health maximally."

"Thus extending the concept of 'managing'?"

"Absolutely! The managers should be individual people, you and me . . . *managing our own health* with the advice and support of physicians and any other people who can contribute. We'll always need high-tech medicine for some things, but it's wrong for everything, and it's a bad substitute for basic, common-sense care of the mind and body. If I could get my patients to eat right, exercise, stop smoking, and deal well with stress, their diabetes would go down, their heart disease would go down, their levels of stress would go down—stress often being a driver or intensifier of other diseases.

"Standard medicine, for what it does, is great. I'm glad we have it. I also like some alternative medicines, for what they do. But the third thing—and in some ways the most basic and most important—is a simple thing, something we might call 'living right.' Heck, we don't even have a name for it, it's so basic and so obvious we can't see it! Furthermore, it runs into political problems with doctors, turf problems, we've-always-done-it-this-way problems, and, of course, economic problems—you can't bill big bucks for *good advice;* it's not a procedure; it's not a money-maker for docs or institutions."

As we walk back to Joe's clinic and the hospital beyond it, I try to picture a lovely modern building with a large sign on it, Good Advice Dispensary, and happy, healthy people going in and out.

That evening, as I drive home, I think of such a dispensary as a kind of utopia: if only we could control all our health factors and live in perfect health for a

very long time. Indeed this concept influences a talk I give for a community
health conference in Missoula. Excited about my topic, I deliver a polemic
about American compulsiveness, speeded-up lifestyles, television ads of sports
utility vehicles driving over glaciers, waterfalls, deserts, and so on. I go on a
tear, ranting against many easy targets. People applaud; there's an article in
the newspaper about my talk—on the front page, no less. I'm thrilled for a day
or two, but I'm not really satisfied, because surely there's something deeper.
Americans' obsessions with wealth, material things, income, and social status
surely rest on more than urges for comfort and ease; I sense a deeper root, an
urge for *control*. I've read that 80 percent of SUV usage is on the roads, going
to work, the grocery store, soccer practices, but the drivers want the feeling that
they could, if necessary, drive over hill and dale, controlling not only nature
but their own fates and destinies. Similarly, undue concern for health and how
we can control it can lead to unhealthy states, as in my hypochondriac games
with my chest pain. Sure, we'd like to control our bodies and live healthy lives
forever, but there are clearly other factors. I think of a brief time I spent in
Morocco, where there's a very different feeling about how much humans can
control; in such an Islamic nation, with prayer five times a day, it is not people
but Allah who is generally assumed to be in control.

An article speaks of a "new world syndrome" in the South Pacific (*Atlantic
Monthly,* June 2001), "a constellation of maladies brought on not by microbes
or parasites but by the assault of rapid Westernization on traditional cultures,"
including diabetes, heart disease, and high blood pressure. Epidemiologists
blame the immediate cause on recent shifts in diet to fatty and salty foods (or
nonfoods), such as sodas, candy bars, potato chips, canned meats, and frozen
turkey tails—all this in a land where native fruits, vegetables, and fish are readily available. An influx of cars and new highways has contributed to less active
lifestyles as well. Many Pacific Islanders are now fat; some have heart attacks
in their twenties; life expectancy is fifty-five. And other similar populations are
affected as well—American Indians, Asian immigrants to wealthy nations—in
short, aboriginal peoples leaving old ways of life for new ones. Geneticists,
however, see a deeper cause than simply the fashionable foods and lowered
physical activity, a "thrifty gene" that converts calories into fat. The theory runs
like this: for thousands of years such peoples lived in marginal conditions and
were subject to floods, droughts, typhoons, and famines. Those who survived
did so because they could store fat better than those who died. Now comes
American/European food, laden with calories, and Polynesians and others very
efficiently pack on the fat. The gene which was once a healthy adaptation is
now a liability. Other cultures with traditionally unstable food supplies (meaning developing nations everywhere) will be at risk for the same problems, the

theory concludes. An interesting conflict looms: educational programs promoting native foods, exercise, and healthy weights versus imported foods with high social value and television showing the "new world," and "labor-saving devices" such as cars. This conflict exists already, of course, in American and Europe. Obesity is now a worldwide epidemic that, paradoxically, can lead to malnourishment when basic nutrients are not included in the huge number of calories consumed. What are public health officials to do? What choices do individuals make? Wherever I go in America, every grocery store has aisles full of sodas and cookies, chips and candies, canned meat, and frozen desserts. There are fruits and vegetables as well, to which our hearts should lead us, but asceticism and perfectionism are not the answers either; indeed, these can be yet another form of stress-causing urges for control.

Following his quadruple bypass operation in 2004, President Bill Clinton became America's most famous heart patient. He now uses his prominence to promote the health of children, specifically through the alliance of his William J. Clinton Foundation with the American Heart Association. In a recent *Parade* magazine article (Sept. 25, 2005), Clinton wrote about the epidemic of childhood obesity in America, urging all of us to help children exercise and eat healthy food.

Besides genetics, other factors are largely outside our control, such as aging, the environment, and accidents both outside and inside of our bodies, factors that will disrupt our lives no matter how well we live. We can't just "be good" and gloat over guarantees we feel we deserve. There are inherent risks in living—accidents, illness, and death—as Michael or Kay can tell us. Maybe living right could put Dr. Knapp out of business, but even living mostly right, most of us will need the help of medicine sooner or later.

My talk about community health led to an invitation to lead a workshop on stress at the university, sponsored by the wellness center there. I resolve to take a less polemical and more realistic approach. Furthermore, what can I learn from the persons who might come?

It's a cool, breezy day as I walk across campus. The sun is high, since it's noon—the only time many faculty are typically free. I make my way to a classroom, carrying my folder of handouts subtly entitled "STOMPING STRESS *** BASHING BURNOUT." (Evidently I still have my own control issues.)

We sit around a rectangle of tables made of handsome blond wood, new and unscarred. I'm confident that the twenty or so folks self-selected to be here are, in fact, stressed—including myself.

"I've got some slips of paper I'm passing around," I say, after introducing myself and our topic. "Would you jot down your three greatest sources of stress, please, and one strategy you have found to combat stress? Let's do this anonymously—no names."

My informants write quickly and pass these back. We do a go-around with names and departments, which shows a good variety across the campus.

"If I can just read through these quickly," I say, and read from the small stack of papers.

"Money, time, work demands."

"Money, job stress, family pressures."

"Not enough time! Money worries, tenure decision looming."

On and on, but finally, "Money! Money! Money!" which draws a good laugh. "Well, one theme is certainly clear."

Over the next hour we talk about stress in general (the word means, at base, pressure or strain, as in stress on architectural structures) and Hans Selye's notions of good stress and bad stress. Some stresses—gravity, air pressure, muscle pull on our bones—are neutral or even good: if we lived with no stress at all, we'd be blobs in some Land of the Lotus-Eaters. We talk about stress in modern America—faster pace of life, competition, specialization, perfectionism, materialism, and repressed emotions, especially anger and sadness. Robert Kugelmann has written a book called *Stress: The Nature and History of Engineered Grief* (Westport, Conn.: Praeger, 1992). He argues the loss of nature (in our cars, our buildings, our cities) causes us grief, which we have turned into pervasive stress. His point may have less weight here in Missoula, perhaps, where many enjoy nature twelve months a year, but the mass media keep fast-paced urban life ever before us as a model. Indeed, most of the professor's strategies for dealing with stress (which I also read out) involve nature: hiking, camping, fishing, skiing, hunting, weekends at a cabin, cooking out in the backyard.

We also talk about pressures specific to our profession (promotion, tenure decisions, relatively low wages for professional work, increasing student loads, publication demands) and our own personal response to such pressures (perfectionism, competition, high motivation, and high ideals). Even the lack of a time clock contributes to stress: we may feel we are never off duty. And we complain about the general lack of reward, recognition, and validation for professional work. Oddly enough, teaching—for all its social components—can be a strangely lonely occupation. Typically we run a class, an entire course by ourselves, and no colleagues ever see how well we do. Students never say, "Great lecture!" or "Gosh, you did a wonderful job marking up my paper!" No registrar ever says, "What a nice set of grades!"

Our discussion turns to coping mechanisms and strategies. Some are clearly negative: alcoholism, depression, anxiety, obsessive behavior, divorce, and suicide, with hypertension and, of course, heart disease being the most common consequences; in their strange, counter-productive ways, these are all methods we use (most often unconsciously) to deal with stress. More positive ways mentioned around the table include using nature as well as hobbies, social groups, worship, exercise, and—in general—activities or states of mind to give feelings of play, being off-duty, being free.

"Just give me a good stream, light tackle, and the prospect of some trout and all my troubles melt away," says one man. As a woman talks about her yoga, her face lights up, and I think of Kay. Maybe I should have called this a "playshop," not a workshop?

We also discuss strategies for dealing with academic life (preparation for promotion and tenure decisions; arranging leaves; social networks beyond departments) and the basic distinction between feeling like a wage-slave ("the help") and feeling like an autonomous professional, regardless of many symbolic messages from our institutions to the contrary.

Finally we talk about blowing off steam, whether with friends, family, a counselor, or more formally through a union, a professional association, even newspapers. Sabotage does not come up, but just knowing that various forms of whistle-blowing are an option—even with inherent risks—helps dilute feelings of victimization and, therefore, stress.

In closing, I say, "If any of you would like to link up today to be 'stress buddies' for the spring semester, say, you could meet by the windows afterwards." No one takes up this particular offer, but I hear lively conversation as people leave.

Driving back to the hospital, I imagine that I haven't told anyone anything new. Newspapers and magazines have been full of articles on stress for a dozen years or more, but nonetheless our culture seems to become more and more stressed. If anything, perhaps I've reminded the professors of specific applications to their professional lives and aspects of self-care that help them (and me) shape emotions and attitudes. In my many years of teaching, I've seen some very unhappy professors, many of whom create unreasonable stresses upon themselves and, regrettably, their colleagues and, even worse, their students. For all their specific knowledge within one field, they are often unaware of some basics in the healthy management—as Dr. Knapp said—of their own lives and in dealing with other human beings.

WHAT STORIES DO WE LIVE? WHAT HABITS OF THE HEART?

Michael's heart defect was congenital, probably the result of embryological malformation; his cardiac dilemmas cannot be explained by his actions or thoughts. His response to his illness, however, is a consciously constructed story he has authored or co-authored, we might say, in collaboration with family, physicians, and other medical helpers. Michael's story includes giving his body over to surgeons for repair. For the operation itself, he's entirely passive, of course, but before and after the operation, he has various future subplots in mind: giving a party with a tape of his heart sounds, getting back on the carousel, physical rehabilitation, including going to Mt. Kilimanjaro with his father. These are positive (or "empowering") stories, because the protagonist (or even hero) of the stories increases in physical power or in affirming emotions, or both. This distinction between raw muscle power and attitude is important, because some sick or dying patients can be healthy in mind and spirit, even though their bodies are failing—something Kay knows a lot about. For Steve, the stories were more on an unconscious level.

There are also disempowering or negative stories available, some of them cultural commonplaces. These can, conversely, diminish our emotional reserves and our physical strength as well. "Life's a bitch, and then you die," reads one bumper sticker. Similarly, "Eat, drink, and be merry, for tomorrow you die" has been the *carpe diem* theme since Roman times. The true Business Stoic welcomes stress, long hours, unreasonable performance goals, and unhealthy office dynamics—the sort of topics currently parodied by the popular cartoon strip "Dilbert." He (or she) is a prime target for marketers of luxury cars, vacations, homes, cigars, clothes—decadent treats surely earned, surely deserved by sacrificial martyrdom. I think a factor in our vulnerability to such advertising is that the stories we live are largely subconscious. We have internalized the basic stories, the myths, the ideologies of our culture so thoroughly that we are not consciously aware of them. Horatio Alger lives, not so much because we read that story any longer but because that story—in many forms—has become part of our culture: *continuous, diligent effort will be richly rewarded!* How many of us as children heard or read *The Little Engine that Could?*

In the last three decades, much thought has been given to the epidemic of heart attacks and the lifestyle choices that the victims have made or at least accepted. The compelling values are embodied in some of our mottoes, such as, *Any boy/girl can grow up to be president, A penny saved is a penny earned, Early to bed and early to rise,* the Darwinian and Spencerian *survival of the fittest,* and so on. *There's only room for one at the top. We are Number One.* The general frenzy of time-urgency, competitiveness, and free-floating anger has been called Type A behavior by cardiologists Meyer Friedman and Ray H. Rosenman in their classic book, *Type A Behavior and Your Heart* (New York: Fawcett Crest, 1974). They describe how a clue to the nervous, hyped-up Type A personalities came from an upholsterer who, assessing chairs in their waiting room, said, "It's so peculiar that only the front edge of your chair seats are worn out." Thinking it over, the doctors realized that their heart patients were anxious, *on the edge of their seats* both physically and psychologically. Such turmoil was typical of their lives; their adrenal systems were overactive, pumping out hormones that scarred their cardiac arteries, thereby inducing the atheromas that would eventually clog those vessels and give them heart attacks. While there has been some debate about this Type A schema, the epidemiological evidence is inescapable: with industrialized lifestyle comes heart disease. Although the causes of heart disease are complex, one area in which individuals can make changes is in their attitudes and behaviors, specifically the stories they choose to live by, the narratives they accept as the guides for their lives. "Heart Attacks Considered Normal in Wall Street" reads a newspaper headline. The story describes how a trader would fall over on the trading floor, while all the rest continued to shout and wave their hands around him to conclude deals. Such an attack, traders said, was simply a risk of their line of work.

Sometimes a dramatic cardiac event, such as Steve's, is the only stimulus strong enough to get our attention, to urge us to rewrite our stories. The new story may include forms of prevention—preventive maintenance, so to speak—an area of American medicine that has been considered less glamorous, less exciting, and less funded than interventive medicine. Our culture loves emergency medicine; we love TV shows based on it. There are no dramatic series during prime time about smoking cessation or eating healthily.

I think of my neighbor back home in Florida, Eddy, who moved in about a year ago. He is often doing some yard work when I walk or jog by in the early morning. We wave or sometimes chat a bit. He's retired from a government job up north. I ask him about his front yard.

"Well, it's coming along. I've removed the plants I needed to and put in half of what I want. The sod's coming next week. Of course, I can only do so much since my heart attack, so I work until I get tired then do some more the next day." He smiles. "After all, I have all the time in the world."

Eddy's calm, cool, and collected; he's an inspiration to me. And I think of other heart patients I have met who are patient and cheerful, as if their heart troubles were a door into a better world. When I visited the Mended Hearts Club meeting at Bayfront Medical Center, for example, I found quite a pleasant group of souls. One man said, "Yep, we're the Zipper Club," pulling up his shirt to show his vertical scar crossed by suture marks. Said another lady, "Well, one thing about having a heart attack is that you realize God has a sense of humor." And she laughed. I realize that this is a self-selected group, since the depressed and/or angry heart patients would not be here (nor even at a Screwed Hearts Club), but people such as Eddy and the Mended Hearts folks exemplify living with limitations, showing that health can include unhealth.

When I visited Cardiac Rehab at the same hospital, I had a similar impression. Most of the patients were elderly and moved slowly. But they seemed to be at peace with themselves. From a rack they'd pick up a small cloth bag with their name on it; a strap went around the neck so that the bag hung on their chests. In the bag went the transmitter that relayed heart rate and blood pressure to a monitor so that one or two nurses could oversee the large room full of exercisers. Patients pedaled on stationary bicycles or walked on treadmills; one cranked with her hands an apparatus much like bike pedals. I saw friendliness not only between patients and staff, but also among patients who greeted each other by name.

Hospital volunteers have made the cloth bags, each with a distinctive color or pattern and a first name written in stitches. Bruce. Carol. Tricia. Bob. Even these bags have symbolic power as gifts of support. The very word "rehabilitation" hinges around the Latin root that means "able," "handy," or "clever," but also "clothing," in the sense of "what fits," being "equipped" or "outfitted." The clothing of our bodies' tissues has been sewn together over millennia; we wear the garments of our skin and hair, but also of our bones, blood, and heart. The psalmist wrote, "For it was you who formed my inward parts; you knit me together in my mother's womb" (Psalms 139:13). Vesalius spoke of the *fabric* of the human body. When our corporeal clothing sustains a rip, physicians, like Dr. Oury, can practice their mending, using their particular instruments. Supportive family and friends also help us to reweave our bodies, help us edit the stories that guide us, the stories we live. The body's warp and woof will eventually unravel, and we need, as well, stories to describe and evaluate such losses. As I consider survivors of cardiac events, I am impressed by persons who have found patience and gratitude to be part of their stories.

When I attended the conference "Medical Applications of Dance, Yoga, and Tai Chi" at the Baylor College of Medicine many years ago, I was struck by a comment one of the speakers made about yoga. He said yoga was intrinsically stress-reducing because the practice relieved individuals of the feeling that they were personally responsible for everything that happened; instead, they were part of—or *sheltered by,* one might say—a world that had its own value and order. When I asked a speaker at an alternative medicine conference what alternative therapies best helped cardiac health, he replied, "Anything that reduces stress."

In their book *Habits of the Heart: Individualism and Commitment in American Life* (Berkeley: Univ. of California Press, 1985), Robert Bellah and his associates wrote about community in a way that suggests that it too can reduce stress on individuals. The title comes from Alexis de Tocqueville, the French visitor to America who studied our *moeurs* (morals), or, in his phrase, "habits of the heart."

In a note, Bellah cites Xavier Zubiri, who believes that Tocqueville, a lifelong student of Pascal, subscribed to some of Pascal's values for the word *heart*. Both saw heart not as sappy sentimentalism but as a kind of commonsense reason that was basic to humans. Bellah writes, "*Heart* in this sense is ultimately biblical. Both the Old and the New Testaments speak of the heart as involving intellect, will, and intention as well as feeling. The notion of 'habits of the heart' perhaps goes back ultimately to the law written in the heart (Deuteronomy 6:6, cf. Jeremiah 31:33, and Romans 2:15). It is interesting that both Confucianism and Buddhism have a notion of the heart that is somewhat comparable." *Habits of the Heart* was much read and commented on in the late 1980s, but its many observations and suggestions seem to have been forgotten since then. Bellah points out, for example, the paradoxical nature of the phrase "private citizen," since none of us can actually live apart from others. And yet our national myths (especially as propagated by the mass media—movies, TV, stories, advertisements) glorify the solitary hero who makes it "on his own"—the cowboy, the hard-boiled detective, the action hero who is typically a loner, a misfit, even a violent man. For Tocqueville, the "habits of the heart" are the notions, opinions, and ideas that "shape mental habits," and "the sum of moral and intellectual dispositions of men [and women] in society." These are not vague abstractions; they have concrete form through "habitual practices" in such areas as religion, political participation, and economic life. In the final chapter, Bellah argues that there is a *counter-story* to the fragmenting and individualizing of America, a story of a culture of coherence that assumes "a morally and intellectually intelligible world"; this story may be promulgated by families, churches, schools, and other organizations. But is it promulgated enough to counter the oppressive stories of the market-driven mass media?

Bellah suggests a "social ecology" through which we all support each other, but it seems we are more likely to act out our own personal versions of the Darwinian survival of the fittest.

A *Washington Post* article speaks of the direct increase of stress in all levels of society when the rich and the poor become further removed from each other. The stress of the poor is easy to grasp: little money, little work, and bad living conditions, often including much crime. But what stresses the rich? The very question seems absurd. And yet people in swanky cars are careful not to drive in "rough" neighborhoods. They lock everything, buy nifty money belts, and live in "gated communities"—another paradoxical phrase—fearing the barbarians without. They're often afraid of losing what they have—typically to the have-nots. And the distance between rich and poor keeps increasing in the United States. (Are we, in fact, "united"? Post–September 11 mottoes speak of standing united, but Republican economic policies still favor the rich.) A recent news report says that some American CEOs make four hundred times the yearly wage of the lowest-paid people in their corporations, a disparity that many cultures (Japan, for example) would consider not only unjust but absurd.

Bellah's "social ecology" assumes a common good, as opposed to what he calls the current "poverty of affluence." (Another movement of social criticism labels the enemy "affluenza.") I think of the multinational corporations that have no home to be responsible to, no home that could offer contextualizing values. Historically, the point of a corporation was to create a legal construct that could go broke without touching the wealth of the managers or directors. And today, a corporation's main purpose is often neither to create a good product, nor to use the world's resources efficiently, nor to offer a service to help society, but rather to increase the earnings per share for the benefit of stockholders (which includes the corporate management and directors). The very word "corporation"—which suggests a *corpus,* a *body*—is ironic, since it is a legal, abstract construct, disembodied from material reality, a neighborhood, the earth, nature, the people who work there, and the people it might serve.

Habits of the Heart is a curious book, bravely analytical and critical of America's weaknesses, yet rationalistic and optimistic in an Enlightenment sort of way that seems to me idealistic to the point of abstraction. The positive focus is on church, social organizations, and political involvement—surely often fine things—but the detailed, nineteen-page index gives no hint of the importance of health or medicine. Further, the authors state that they have primarily studied the white middle class, a weakness that limits the application of this research to a multicultural society. And the rational world the book promotes has no room for transcendence, mystery, or even "acts of God" that will inevitably try us all. But beyond these reservations, I like the emphasis on society as a source of *heartedness,* a reducer of stress, a way to live in peace. I am confident that if the book's ideals were adopted at least in part, there would be less heart illness in America.

One weekend my wife and I are driving up the Clark Fork to go hiking. She has studied the Bellah volume, and we are discussing it. As we drive along a cut in a hillside that the waters of the Clark Fork began millennia ago and that highway engineers extended some decades ago, we see many layers of ancient seabed compressed into rock, then wrinkled and uplifted into the Rocky Mountains. Nancy says, "I wonder what Bellah would say about that." I wonder too. As I review the book later, it seems to me that he and his colleagues have concentrated on *human* nature, seeing it in Cartesian fashion as separate from *nature* nature, the geophysical world around us, and a source of heartedness. (I think of Gretchen Ehrlich's criticism that we don't pay attention to nature because we don't attend to our bodies; perhaps the reverse is equally true.) Once again, the earth-nurtured Antaeus comes to mind; are we strangling ourselves with stress as we dangle above the earth?

YELLOWSTONE

My wife Nancy has suggested several times that we drive down from Missoula to Yellowstone National Park. Somehow I haven't become excited because I've been there twice before, first as a youth and later when she and I were newlyweds. When we camped there in the 1960s, one of the high points was the capture of a marauding bear not far from our tent. We had been warned against having any food left out or in our tent and against wearing any hair oil. About 11:00 P.M. there was a loud clang, and we campers converged, wearing pajamas and carrying flashlights, to look into the trap, a fifty-five-gallon drum baited with bacon fat. It was hard to make out anything amidst the shadows and the dark fur that filled the drum, but soon we could see two black eyes peering back at us, expressionless. Although the canvas walls of our tent still seemed awfully thin, we all slept better that night in that land of primal forces.

And now suddenly it's some thirty years later and I feel there's plenty to see on weekends right around Missoula. Besides, we've been driving a rented car, a dinky, under-powered thing that struggles up mountain passes. We're scheduled to have a better car once all the tourists leave, but that will be later in the fall, when going to Yellowstone would be risky because of snow on the high passes, not to mention in Yellowstone itself, which is mostly above seven thousand feet. Although the drive to Yellowstone is some 250 miles over several mountain ranges including the Continental Divide, I know, at some deep, intuitive level, that my wife is right: we really must go. When someone mentions a good place to stay in the Paradise Valley just north of the park, the last of my resistance crumbles, and we drive down from Missoula, approaching Yellowstone from the north.

Yellowstone was the first national park anywhere on the globe, and is still the largest. Tourists come from all over the world to see the scenery, the geothermal wonders, and the wildlife. The tourist guides say that it is the largest center of geothermal activity on earth (more than in Iceland, even) and a continuing experiment in animal and land management. The large wild herd of bison has been rebuilt from numbers as small as twenty-five. Deer, elk, moose, bear, and mountain goats roam freely, not to mention foxes, martins, muskrats, ground squirrels, otters, chipmunks, and the newly reintroduced gray wolves from Canada.

What is less well known—and what I never heard in two visits before—is that Yellowstone Park is the remains of a gigantic volcano, perhaps the largest ever to exist on earth. It blew its top about 600,000 years ago in an explosion that sent rocks, ash, soil, lava, and cinders over about two thirds of the current forty-eight contiguous states, an amount of material calculated to have been about six hundred times larger than the material spectacularly blown out of Oregon's Mt. St. Helens in 1980! The Ur-Yellowstone Mountain must have been an immense mountain, bigger than Shasta, bigger than Hood, bigger than Rainier, to pick some of the lovely conical mountains of the Pacific Cascades. I've seen Mt. St. Helens from the air, easily spotting the northern side that blew out, leaving the rough shape of an enormous armchair. At Yellowstone, however, the *entire* cone blew up, leaving bits of rim in a large, irregular circle. Some remnants fell back into the cavern below, creating an inner floor that comprises much of the park today. A ranger explained this primal story to us at Old Faithful, pointing to a section of the rim directly to the west. *Good Lord,* I thought, *we're standing in the barrel of a volcanic gun.* The technical term for such a crater is *caldera* (literally, a warm or hot pot, as in the word *cauldron*). Thus Yellowstone Lake is similar in geologic form to Crater Lake, although not so circularly neat. Where the lake spills over the northern edge of the caldera, we have the magnificent Upper Falls of the Yellowstone River, which has continued for millennia to excavate the Grand Canyon of the Yellowstone. Here visitors peer down a thousand feet into a V-shaped canyon of variegated beiges, tans, oranges, and of course yellows—for which the river and the park are named.

The geothermal effects loved by visitors include the famous geysers, the clownish mud pots, the hissing and steaming fumaroles, and the hot springs. All of these are powered by hot water straight below us, in a complex system of tunnels that extends two miles down to the heat source, a bubble of magma, molten rock which is ordinarily much deeper in the earth. (One speculation suggests that a meteorite caused this rogue bubble, a theory that I like for its cosmic scope.) Yellowstone, like the western coast of the United States, has had many earthquakes of many sizes and durations. And, yes, the volcano beneath our feet as we walk the boardwalks to see the sights, the volcano we are walking on—or *in*—is still alive. Since it's reckoned to blast every 600,000 years, it could go any minute. More likely, it will go sometime in the next 100,000 years—a calming thought. But the stark truth is that to visit Yellowstone—having ice cream, walking beside the boiling water, strolling through the Old Faithful Inn—is to lollygag atop a temporary plug in a mammoth piece of artillery. Someday it'll all be shot into the skies once again.

As you drive to the Park, you may not notice a climb, but you gain 2,000 to 3,000 feet to reach any of the five entrances. These approaches are, of course, the lower slopes of the former volcano. When you drive up onto the floor of the crater, you're at 7,367 feet at Old Faithful. To the southwest, there's an 8,500 foot knob. In every other direction there are 10,000-foot mountains. In one sense it's the top of the local world, since the Continental Divide runs through it, separating the Pacific and the Mississippi drainages. Indeed, four river systems exit from the Park—much like the biblical Eden or the mythic geography of the ancient historian Paulus Orosius. The Snake River flows south to the Tetons, then west across lava fields to join the Columbia on the way to the Pacific; the Gallatin goes northwest to become part of the headwaters of the Missouri, which flows into the Mississippi, which goes to New Orleans (the Missouri-Mississippi drainage is second only to the Amazon drainage in South America); to the north is the Yellowstone, which will join the Missouri as far away as North Dakota; and to the east, the Shoshone, which will join the Yellowstone in Montana. Both geysers and snowmelt supply these rivers, as does, of course, rain.

The word "entrance" carries the usual sense of entry, but also, in this case, the sense of *trance,* the mental state induced by hypnosis or magic. The land—once you get there, once you start to *pay attention*—takes you out of your ordinary consciousness: truly this is a place of primal origins, a place to see, smell, hear, and feel the story of land and to live among wildlife that has lived here longer than humans have existed. Along the Lamar Valley in the north part of the park are some of the most ancient rocks known, so-called basement rocks, reckoned by radiocarbon dating to be 2.7 billion years old. The outflow streams from the hot springs are multicolored, owing to bacteria living there, their colors corresponding to the intensity of the heat. Scientists believe that studying them may help us to understand the origins of all life on this planet, since similar bacteria may have grown in the hot waters formed by the first rains on the hot surfaces of the earth. And still, rocks are being formed, such as travertine along the ridges of the Mammoth Hot Springs. Beneath our feet and all around us lies an entire scale of geologic time and its wonders.

But we are hardly the first to enjoy this place. For some nine thousand years American Indians had this land to themselves. They came for plentiful game, retreating during the harsh winters. (Wildlife tends to stay year-round, moving from higher to lower elevations for the winters because of the geothermal heat and the well-watered vegetation.) It's certainly possible that these grounds were holy to some tribes. Even in economic-utilitarian terms, the obsidian cliffs were prized for their black, semi-transparent stone, which could be made into blades, axes, and arrow points. The geological explanation of obsidian gives me chills: hot lava erupting from below, intersected with the glacier above and crystallized into glass.

Living in cities or traveling in placid landscapes dulls our sense of the earth's dynamic history. At Yellowstone our imaginations, our feelings wake up to space and time through the dramatic imagery of boiling geysers, large canyons, and high mountains. The Romantics called these sensations "the sublime," meaning the entrancement, the awe, even the fear we feel when confronting overwhelming stimuli. The young Edmund Burke wrote a treatise on the sublime and the beautiful, preferring the sublime to the merely neat and pretty. Modern Americans are so used to the special effects of movies, violence, and other extreme events, it's hard for them to feel any sense of the sublime, except perhaps through drugs, sex, high-risk sports, or . . . nature.

Not five minutes after arriving in the park, our car is stopped by a herd of elk crossing the road. The bull stops to raise his head and bugle, a long yodeling call that raises the hair on the back of my neck. That afternoon three hundred bison, their heads hung low from massive shoulders, cross the road and surround our halted car at their own deliberate pace. Our car feels flimsy. A bull bison could easily upturn it.

Yellowstone is a place where we can get perspective, see ourselves among large beasts, natural forces, geologic time. When we see signs warning about falling a thousand feet into the Grand Canyon of the Yellowstone, or being gored by bison, or boiling to death in the hot springs, we think about violent yet natural death. Here and there we see bleaching bones of large creatures who broke through crusts around hot spots and died there. Park policy is to leave the bones there to show nature at work. (In a death-aversive culture, it is good to be reminded of mortality.) Similarly, the forest fires of 1988 were a lesson in destruction and renewal; ten years later, a myriad of small lodgepole pines carpet the burned areas. The prescriptive lessons of Smokey the Bear have been superseded by an understanding that suppressing all fires makes forests more dangerous as fuels build up. Fires also renew minerals in the soil and allow for open areas where sun and precipitation can work. The regrowing areas of Yellowstone are now vital, rich with vegetation and wildlife. In a linear culture, it is good to see cycles, however long, at work. The subterranean magma that powers Yellowstone is an analogue to the blood in our arteries and veins. The magma carries minerals and other nutrients to the various parts of the earth, destroying and also creating. Its cousin, boiling water, pumps back and forth in the chambers below the park, a cyclical pulse of both water and heat that makes life—whether bacterial or mammalian—possible. The outer layer of the earth, the skin we live on, demonstrates a circulatory dynamism at many speeds, from the explosions of volcanoes to the slow, slow processes of erosion and tectonic plates' migration. As *The Epic of Gilgamesh* put it some five thousand years ago, change is the law of life.

Trying to learn from the park and manage it in ways that work with nature have been challenges over the last hundred years, and rangers increasingly take their cues from the way this area has always managed itself. The notion that nature has its own intelligence is the basis for the Gaia hypothesis proposed by scientists James Lovelock and Lynn Margulis. According to this view, the earth's intelligence can, for example, keep ocean salinity stable over centuries despite many variables; while many scientists are reluctant to anthropomorphize the earth this way, the hypothesis raises good questions. Is an aggregate of forces an intelligence, or just an accumulation of random events? Does it matter whether humans understand all the factors? After all, the human body works quite well despite our ignorance of many of its functions. To visit Yellowstone is to renew our sense that nature *works,* whether in rocks, trees, or in cardiac tissue. Or perhaps the Gaia (or Gaea) hypothesis says more about humans than about nature: we want a spirit of place, a female spirit; we want an earthly home that has a tempering intelligence. Antaeus-like, we want to touch our mother earth and receive nurturing power.

Nancy and I went in mid-September, a good time (we thought) to have the park to ourselves, since children would be back in school, and their parents back at work to pay for the summer vacations. Those people weren't there, but everyone else was: retired people, singles, bikers, traveling Asians, Europeans—you name them. Parking lots were mostly full. Along with maybe five hundred other people, we watched Old Faithful blast over one hundred feet into the sky. When the wind shifted, warm water fell on us, and people scattered one way or another. Fortunately the superheated water had cooled in the air, so the spray felt more like a baptism or a kiss than a geothermic attack, and I heard around me laughter and joyful cries.

ENJOYING CHAOS MORE

In his church office, Steve and I continue our conversation about his angina pectoris.

"As things moved on, there were still some rough spots. We couldn't eat at our favorite restaurants because of my diet. Hell, the diet didn't even appear to be working for six months. Brenda even put up with the cabin I suddenly, impulsively, bought outside of town. It was irrational ... and I spent hours up there fixing it up. Now I know I was picking up pieces and reassembling them, both the cabin and my life. I wanted a *nest* ... I wanted to stay in Missoula and have roots. In a strange sort of way I could understand the survivalists, those guys stockpiling stuff out in the woods. I got an old car and fixed it up." This is a 1939 Plymouth coupe—bright purple. It's well known in town, contrasting vividly with the pickups and sports utility vehicles.

"I started to write blues songs, poems." In earlier years, Steve had been a blues musician. "I love the blues tradition. It comes from poor people, beaten down blacks in particular, who put words to feelings of loss. Sometimes it's only an oppressed people who can see reality, the Jungian shadow stuff we usually deny. I was re-accessing feelings and intuitions I had lost. I had to start out introspectively and work my way outwards. At base, it's all about connectedness, belonging, and meaning."

He pauses to look out the window. I know he loves this church and its grounds. For All Saints' Day he suggested that parishioners dress up in costumes for Sunday worship, but the choir (in which my wife and I sing) was not excited by this idea. After all, this was an Episcopal church, and a rather formal one at that. We singers wore red robes with white surplices over them and a chain and cross over that. We finally compromised on a minimal gesture, haloes on our heads. Much of the rest of the congregation, however, pitched in with all sorts of costumes. One man wore a huge miter and full ecclesiastical regalia. In the service Steve asked him whether he was a bishop or the Pope, and everyone laughed. As the congregation came up for communion at the rail, the choir in the chancel watched all the wonderful costumes. Steve's loony idea had worked.

When a new slate roof was nearing completion, Steve was conversing with one of the craftsmen, an Indian who said that he was a medicine man for his tribe. Further, he offered to help Steve bless the roof, and Steve accepted. (I think many ministers would not have been so ecumenical.) Accordingly, both men rode a hydraulic bucket to the edge of the roof then climbed up a ladder lying on the sharp pitch. With due care, they made their way to the concrete cross at the intersection of the nave and the two transepts. In church talk, this is the crossing, a central, unifying point; in some European cathedrals there's a particular tile design, a labyrinth, for example, on the floor below. In Missoula, Montana, we had an Anglo minister and an Indian holy man riding the roof ridge, saying prayers and leaving symbols tucked into the cross some sixty feet above the ground. The next Sunday, when the congregation heard about this ceremony, we felt doubly blessed.

Steve continues. "I gave up the old time-urgency ways ... deadlines ... the *should-ought-must* stuff I had been taught. I'm now enjoying chaos more. There are surprises, things that come toward you, things you'd never expect. And ... if you're too goal-oriented, you'll never see them.

"I'm eleven years out now from the plumbing of my heart and haven't had to go back. In an ironic way, the sickness healed me. In some ways, I got better. In other ways, I'm just the same ... only I know better who I am and that it's OK to be limited, to be mortal."

"Sickness, in some sense, healed you?"

"Yes. It gets you out of the lie we live here in America."

"The lie?"

"That everything must be perfect."

"A case of the perfect being the enemy of the good?"

"Truly."

"How's the cholesterol?" I ask.

"Oh, we're down to 150. I got down to 280 through diet and exercise. It took a drug to pull it down to 150, but I've held it there—again, diet and exercise—for five years now, without medicines. I don't eat red meat, cheese, or eggs. Motivation has been easy: I did not want to live the life of a heart patient, disabled for the rest of my life. I do fast walking for forty-eight minutes four times a week. In the summer I work on raising trees out by my cabin. I try to stay mellow."

"What about the spiritual side . . . being a priest and all?"

"Ha! You should have heard one of my docs. He said, 'With all those smart Episcopal lawyers in your flock, you should wangle a snazzy disability buyout.' Can you imagine? I loved my work. I felt I was just getting started here. I couldn't give that up.

"What I felt was a giant *disconnect* from the rest of the world. I'd see people on the street going about their regular lives and think, *Idiots . . . don't they know?* I was feeling deep grief, a total loss of meaning . . . my life might be over all too soon. I fell back on a childlike faith and trust that God would lead me to *higher ground*. I got that phrase from a friend . . . you know, as if I were drowning. And whatever higher ground might mean: healing, a merciful death, or a better acceptance of my illness."

"Did your prayer life change?"

"Not really . . . I've never been a morning prayer person. Although . . . yes, in a way it did, because I started saying a mantra I made up:

Live each day to the fullest
    For the joy that is in it.
Embrace the sorrows, the chances,
    And changes in the world in which we live.
Love Brenda.
Be kind.

"That's it."

"How often did you say that?"

"One hundred times a day. That and books and blues really helped see me through. And friends. And medicine. And grace. After all, if I hadn't tried to lift that piano, I might well be dead now. I'll be dead someday, of course, but I'm so glad I got a second life first."

Solid Footing, Higher Ground (Third Essay)

The Rocky Mountains are massive and uncompromising. Looking down a valley lined on both sides with crags and glaciers makes me aware of my tiny stature but expands my imagination. As I drive along the Clark Fork, I think about the man it was named for, William Clark, one of the first white men through here, and his journey with Lewis on their way to the Pacific Ocean roughly two centuries ago. In the cuts of the river, I see layers of sedimentary rock laid down over the immense time spans, when a huge inland sea covered the middle of today's America and Canada. These layers are usually tipped up on an angle, as the earth's crust moved, cracked upward, twisted, waved, bulged, or dived—slow motion gymnastics neatly shown in museums and geology books. (Even Mount Everest has seafloor for a peak.) The hours and years of my life are, again, as nothing against a geologic scale of time; the Yellowstone volcano went off some 600,000 years ago and is due "now." Indeed, these mountains are as dangerous as they are beautiful. You can't live out here and not pay attention to the weather, proper clothing, tires, and adequate supplies in your house for a three-day blizzard. This environment helps keep people healthy; they can see—indeed must see—the larger picture. For outdoor enthusiasts, many factors are important. The parasite giardia is in many streams; therefore, you carry your own water (or a superb filter), as well as your food. Temperatures can change quickly. It's wise to hike with a buddy, in case of a sprained ankle. Many people carry pepper spray against a bear or cat attack. Nature and human nature—how do we best fit in? What social links—starting with a hiking companion—support us and our hearts?

"Living out here is a blood sport," Nancy remarks one day as we're hiking in a chilly gorge. We were on this same trail earlier in the fall, when the sun shone directly on our path. Now, lower in a late autumn sky, the sun doesn't reach us. There's ice along the side of the stream. If you are not careful—or gravely unlucky—you can get frozen, eaten, or shot. You can die of hypothermia or dehydration. You can drink alcohol and tumble out of a boat or fall off a cliff. About once a week there's such a story in the newspaper.

Most fall weekends in Montana found my wife and me hiking, guided by a paperback that described day hikes around Missoula. This document would have been enough, but I insisted on getting the topographical maps that showed features in wonderful detail. A Florida flatlander, I particularly enjoyed the elevation contours; I'd calculate the length of our hike and its vertical climb. I was the big-picture quester, the Point A to Point B strategist, measuring by watch and compass. (Indeed, the magazine ads for a watch that included a barometer, an altimeter, and a thermometer briefly tempted me.) I found large natural features, directions, the lay of the land with ease. As I reflected on these urges, they seemed to be remnants of the urban world I was used to, where strategies of control were rewarded. One of my previous hobbies was running, with a full season of races, during which we'd charge through parks, beaches, and neighborhoods seeing little of what was there, but hitting our mile markers according to plan. Even in the Rockies, obsessed with linear pursuits, I strode past many an interesting feature that my wife would call me back to: an animal track, a ground squirrel behind a tree, or a tiny, alpine wildflower. I slowly accommodated my approach to the nature-hike model, which allowed, if I was patient, more details to come to me. Issues of control slowly became opportunities for serendipity or grace, and my love of nature grew. E. O. Wilson speaks of "biophilia," a love for biological forms that is a deep instinct in humans. The word "ecology" is based on a Greek root for "house," a place where we feel at home, as in Steve's sense of a nest, his cabin in the woods.

Up one of the ravines of the Bitterroot (at about 4,500 feet), we stopped to sit on some boulders in the middle of an icy stream and eat our sandwiches. In a while Nancy said, "Hey, look at that," pointing to a small, comical, dark bird that was bobbing in the water below us. Having read John Muir's ecstatic essay, she recognized it as a dipper or water ouzel. The ouzel worked its way upstream, looking for whatever it is that ouzels eat. We stayed still and watched him maneuver over rocks and freshets, precise and balletic. He came within ten feet of us and passed on upstream. His lunch and ours . . . his activity and our inactivity, his heart beating away quickly under load and ours beating slowly at rest. At a nature class we attended, the instructor suggested that people sit in one place for an hour as the best way to see wildlife. "Unless they smell you, they won't know you're there." You can hear the call of the wild on a dramatic trip through Yellowstone or sitting still on a rock in a stream or even spending some time in an urban yard as birds, clouds, and insects pass by.

For anyone who loves nature, Montana is a land of staggering beauty. High clouds sail by overhead . . . sunsets are often wonderful . . . the lower mountains have massive shoulders with fringes of dark forests, especially Douglas firs and Ponderosa pines. (If you put your nose to a Ponderosa on a warm day, you smell a sweet vanilla.) Ground squirrels and other rodents scamper about. We've seen a pileated woodpecker twenty feet away. Streams flow down the ravines with little falls, cascades, and braided sections. Pools big enough for wading are chilly, often shaded, often fed by snow melt. On a bird walk, we saw an ornithologist call a hawk across the Bitteroot River to a tree near us. Big birds cruise overhead, hawks, bald eagles, golden eagles. They can see a mouse half a mile away. The higher mountains are of every shape: knife edge, spire, upraised slab with a jagged edge. Squaw Peak, visible from Missoula, is an extinct volcano, a perfect cone.

The water ouzel, the deer, the golden eagles, the cutthroat trout—and even humans—all these have hearts designed exactly for the particular lives of each species. The human heart has been designed for activity, a dynamic life, but—equally important—also for rest and renewal. As Steve found, unrelieved stress is dangerous to the heart. He had to study the subconscious stories—those deeply embedded in our culture—that drove his behavior, bring these to consciousness, and rewrite them. His new story domesticated him with this Montana valley; he reconnected himself to nature with his cabin and his tree farm. He created a mantra, words that guide his thinking by values he consciously chose, not the subconscious and unhealthy values of overachievement, perfection, illusions of personal control. Some wonderful combination of his medical treatment and his own changes in thought and behavior brought about a healing of his heart.

Steve was lucky. Not all patients (heart or otherwise) profit from excellent care and the results of their own personal changes. Indeed, one troubling aspect of alternative medicine, new age medicine, even Dr. Knapp's "living right" is that they suggest that we have absolute control over our lives, our health, our destinies. Patients who believe that mind-over-matter can cure them are often disappointed when they don't get well as fast as they'd like or when they don't get well at all. Efforts at stress reduction can become a substitute obsession, another form of stress.

Like the genetic backgrounds of obesity we looked at earlier, the behavioral dimensions of health are also complex, even though, in theory, they appear readily controllable. I remember a drug educator speaking to my students. She had an effective rhetorical device: "Imagine that you could have any car you wanted, but that it was the only car you'd have forever. What kind of gas would you put into it? How often would you have it serviced?" And so on. When she had the students well hooked, she suggested that car was a metaphor for the human body and that people typically took better care of their cars than of their bodies. While arresting and inspiring, the comparison suggests that we have complete control over our cars and our bodies, as if impervious to disease and accidents. I think of the Polynesians and their propensity to gain weight and, by contrast, the Russian skater Sergei Grinkov who died of a sudden heart attack while on the ice for a practice session. Winner of many championships and two Olympic gold medals, he was surely in superb shape, with none of the usual behavioral risk factors for heart illness (smoking, diabetes, old age, sedentary lifestyle, high blood pressure, or high cholesterol). Johns Hopkins scientist Pascal Goldschmidt believes that a variant gene may have been a crucial factor.

An article in the *American Journal of Public Heath* describes an elaborate effort over thirteen years, the Minnesota Heart Health Program, then the largest of its kind, with some 400,000 persons. This was an intense program of interviews, lab work, counseling of individuals, groups, and communities at large, mass media education, and school-based health promotion programs. The results, however, were modest. In their words, "Many intervention components proved effective in targeted groups. However, against a background of strong secular trends of increasing health promotion and declining risk factors, the overall program results were modest in size and duration and generally within chance levels" (84.9: 1383). Any statistics showing improved health in general are, of course, good, but beating an average by raising an entire population is difficult. Programs focused for particular groups worked the best, but, once again, absolute control—even with the best techniques and method—seem to elude us.

While good advice about health is readily available in the mass media, many people persist in "poor health habits," often for compelling reasons. I spoke with a pulmonologist in North Carolina, a state that raises huge amounts of tobacco, a product that impacts health on a large scale, especially the lungs and the heart. She said, "We can control nicotine with pills and patches pretty well now, but that's not the only factor. People get used to smoking as a ritual, as a reward, as something they can count on in their lives. For some people, smoking is like another member of the family." People working stressful jobs, commuting, and dealing with a crowded, noisy neighborhood cannot en masse move to the mountains. (Some do, of course, sometimes bringing their stressed lifestyles with them.) Stress reduction, for all my good advice to the faculty workshop, seems to work best as a series of individual choices.

Because the heart cannot be seen in an absolute, objective way, considerations of the heart lead eventually to how we exist in the world, or who we are. It is our eyes, our expectations, and other lenses through which we see the heart that become crucial, whether scientific or humanistic, or both. Our views of nature are influenced by our own human nature. One famous exposition of humans' complexity is a dialogue between the heart and the head, written by Thomas Jefferson in 1786. About ten pages long, it's the bulk of a letter to Maria Cosway, a British painter whom Jefferson knew during his Paris years. Biographers are not sure whether there was an actual affair, but clearly there were strong emotions between the two, who admired the sights of Paris together. The occasion is Maria's departure to England and Jefferson's first letter to her. In the dialogue, the Head speaks rationally, upbraiding the Heart for its follies and excesses, and affirming that "Everything in this world is a matter of calculation." The Heart—bewailing its grief in exaggerated, lyrical language studded with exclamation points—rejects such "miserable arithmetic" and "frigid speculations," concluding:

When nature assigned us the same habitation, she gave us over it a divided empire. To you she allotted the field of science, to me that of morals. When the circle is to be squared, or the orbit of a comet to be traced; when the arch of greatest strength, or the solid of least resistance is to be investigated, take you the problem; it is yours: nature has give me no cognisance of it. In like manner in denying to you the feelings of sympathy, of benevolence, of gratitude, of justice, of love, of friendship, she has excluded you from their control. To these she has adapted the mechanism of the heart.

We have here a precursor of C. P. Snow's s two cultures, reason versus emotion, a conflict that appears in many novels and plays, as far back as Sophocles' *Antigone*. We even continue the division today, testing our youth according to verbal or mathematical skills. But aren't some of the wisest, happiest people those who can integrate their heads and their hearts? I've known plenty of passionate scientists . . . and plenty of analytic humanists.

I have more and more respect for bosses, middle managers, even high-level administrators who encourage a healthy workplace, and for anyone who maintains good relationships with other people at work and elsewhere. I've seen offices with comfortable furniture, full-spectrum lighting, pleasant colors, art on the walls, easy passage around workstations, and areas for relaxation and chance conversations that may deepen social ties or even lead to imaginative thinking about work. Two thousand hours at work—or roughly one-third of our waking hours—per year should, ideally, be under good conditions. And what about our neighborhoods, our schools, our play areas for children and adults? How can we provide for the full-spectrum needs of human nature, both the head and the heart? How can we link the ground—or sidewalks or floors—under our feet with the most abstract thoughts of our minds? Where can we find solid footing *and* higher ground?

My search for the heart has taken me to different hospitals, labs, libraries, and informants. But, like the experience with the water ouzel, sometimes it's waiting and listening that bring the heart to us. One evening I asked Nancy if I could listen to her heart—but my stethoscope was some three thousand miles away. After a few awkward attempts, we found it easiest for her to lie on our bed, for me to place my ear on her sternum. I quieted my mind and heard her heart beating, the famous *lub dub* with a rest, then again . . . and again. The first pitch was lower and duller, the second a higher pitch and more vibrant—a bass drum followed by a small kettle drum. With each of her breaths the heart speeded up a little then slowed down. "Gosh," I said, "Your heart really sounds like it knows what it's doing." She said, "Let me hear yours," and we changed positions. As her head settled on my chest, my arms draped around her head and shoulders. I liked the intimate position, as for nursing a baby. We were close, caring. I felt no hurry to move. Eventually she looked up at me and smiled, "Yeah . . . it's really loud. It sounds powerful."

The twinges I was feeling in my chest at the beginning of our Montana stay are now gone. One reason, I think, was my wife's voice as she listened to my heart and said it was strong. Her voice has replaced the little paranoid voice I was harboring, teasing myself, making life interesting by imagining the worst case for my heart. Another reason is a less stressful life here in the mountains, as opposed to the urban, crowded life in Florida with my usual load of classes, committees, and campus politics. But I shouldn't just blame my environment; ultimately it's my own response that makes them stressful or not.

Now I can perceive my heart with a new heritage, a pedigree of millions of years that created it, the miraculous fetal development that grew it, and its place within the immense frameworks of nature, both in time and in space. Our hearts are part of nature, the animal world, the geological world, the huge dimensions of time and space the Rockies display. Our hearts are made of the same basic elements as much of the natural world—hydrogen, carbon, nitrogen, and oxygen—whether in the soil underfoot or the stars as far as we can see. Our hearts are part of the powers of nature dramatically shown at Yellowstone, powers that are active in farms and cities, even along interstate highways—wherever we go. Wherever we live, we can't really leave nature, except in our forgetfulness of it, our denial of it.

The old story of my heart was the pump that would break, the clock that would run down, the assassin waiting in ambush. The new story is that the human heart is a gift of nature, a wonder, a rare and ingenious organ created from materials of the universe—custom-made for each one of us. But the heart is vulnerable to stresses, as we live within a larger society. What Steve shows me is that we can bring the hidden, implicit stories that control us into consciousness so that we can either edit them or replace them with new, consciously affirmed stories that guide and support us. Such stories, even in all their verbal vaporousness, can provide both a higher ground and a solid footing. As in Jefferson's notion of a dialogue, another metaphor for the heart, it seems to me, is *partner*. From our birth to our death we are partnered with our hearts. Our hearts, perhaps blindly, perhaps dumbly, but nonetheless relentlessly, keep our blood flowing for as long as we live.

Alcove Model: Three Perspectives on the Heart

a. Person

b. A biological definition of heart

c. Diagnosed illness(es)

d. Branch of treating medicine

e. Medical intervention(s)

f. Patient concept(s) of heart

g. Patient support strategies

h. Humanistic perspective

i. Outcome aim

j. Exemplary metaphor

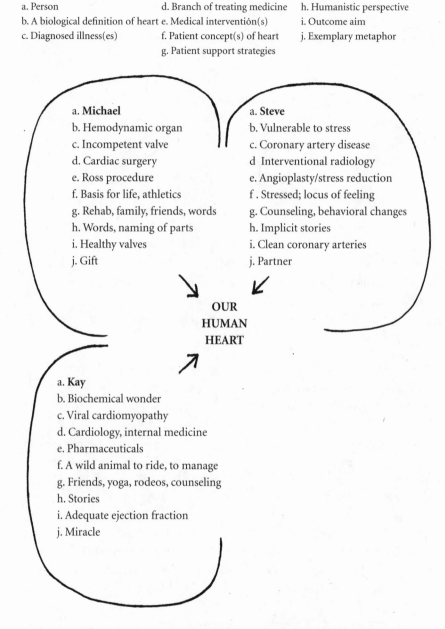

a. **Michael**

b. Hemodynamic organ

c. Incompetent valve

d. Cardiac surgery

e. Ross procedure

f. Basis for life, athletics

g. Rehab, family, friends, words

h. Words, naming of parts

i. Healthy valves

j. Gift

a. **Steve**

b. Vulnerable to stress

c. Coronary artery disease

d Interventional radiology

e. Angioplasty/stress reduction

f . Stressed; locus of feeling

g. Counseling, behavioral changes

h. Implicit stories

i. Clean coronary arteries

j. Partner

OUR HUMAN HEART

a. **Kay**

b. Biochemical wonder

c. Viral cardiomyopathy

d. Cardiology, internal medicine

e. Pharmaceuticals

f. A wild animal to ride, to manage

g. Friends, yoga, rodeos, counseling

h. Stories

i. Adequate ejection fraction

j. Miracle

Alcove Model showing three perspectives of the heart. Steve's experience illustrates a psychosocial, behavioral, or epidemiological view of the heart.

Johnnie and Zelma Reddick
and the Heart's Reasons

IMAGES AND THE INEFFABLE

Across the street from my former home in Florida lives Bill Parsons, who is a scholar of Russian history. Bill and his wife Vivian taught at the same college for many years with me and my wife, and we all shared various interests in history, literature, and the arts. One day I admired a small painting, a portrait by their front door, Byzantine, it seemed. I asked about it.

"Well," said Bill, "it's an icon, of course, a stylized picture of a saint. The eyes are the main thing. They're like a supernatural channel."

"Hmm, you mean bringing heaven to earth?"

"Oh, at least. It works the other way too for believers, a kind of a portal into the world beyond as you contemplate the image."

"So the image works both ways."

"Yes, but it's hard to put into language. If you have that faith, the connection is immediate and beyond words."

"Ineffable."

"Yes, ineffable, but here we are talking about it," Bill chuckled.

It's a paradox, of course, that language can only go so far but that we keep returning to it as one of our best media for information, persuasion, entertainment, and exploration of the mind. I heartily believe in music, art, dance, touch, and other nonverbal forms of experience, but I also believe in the dialectic of each of them with language that describes and otherwise probes them and their meanings. An image such as the Byzantine icon holds many meanings, including meanings that vary with the viewer's beliefs and expectations. In the dialectic between image and the imagination of the viewer, there can be many levels, meanings that are beyond words, meanings that words can only point to, and meanings that readily translate into words. There can be compressed stories implied by an image, stories of hope or despair.

Upon my return to Florida from Montana, I sensed a gap in my research. My three informants so far were all white, professional people all under fifty-five years of age. I needed to widen my scope. A few phone calls put me in touch with Johnnie and Zelma Reddick, who agreed to talk with me. Although the Reddicks believe in standard western medicine and have used it for Johnnie's various heart ailments, and although Zelma is a registered nurse, they also believe in approaches from alternative medicine, including prayer and a deeply spiritual life. "Alternative medicine" is a modern term that includes many kinds of medicine practiced as folk medicine for millennia before the rise of Western medicine, and many people, especially indigenous peoples, still follow folk beliefs. Furthermore, many westerners—doctors included—often use "alternative" practices, such as massage, imagery, meditation, diet manipulations, and prayer. Estimates for patient usage go as high as 50 percent. Standard medicine ignored all this for much of the twentieth century but then decided that the term "complementary and alternative medicine," or CAM, might define a new, productive relationship between the two. The National Institutes of Health (available on the Internet) is now conducting a series of studies under this CAM rubric to explore the efficacy of specific practices as well as their interactions—positive, neutral, or negative—with standard medicine. I hope they do find scientific evidence that will help traditional physicians talk to their patients about complementary treatment or even to deliver it themselves. I also imagine that some factors (placebo response, for example) will be hard to define, and that some feelings of well-being among patients will be—once again—ineffable.

One factor in a patient's psychological state is a sense of being nurtured, or nourished; even the word "nurse" is a related word and concept. We remember being sick as children and being cared for, cosseted by our mothers. In my family there was the ritual of loading the family dog onto the bed of the patient under the title of "Nurse Ben." Did we heal from our colds any more quickly attended by such a loving beast? Could multicenter, double-blind studies show efficacy? I don't know, but I will claim that being ill while being well nurtured is, at the very least, a more pleasant experience than being ill while feeling lonely and blue.

SKIP SOMETHING . . . SHE RAISES HELL

I pull up to the Reddicks' house in St. Petersburg, Florida, at 3:00 P.M. on a hot, steamy Monday afternoon. I got their names from Rev. Fred Terry, whose church they attend. When I spoke with Zelma Reddick on the phone, I said that I didn't want a book about hearts with just white folks in it. She said, "Yes, we get heart disease too . . . and at a higher rate than white people."

The house and yard are meticulously cared for. All the bushes are trimmed; the lawn is edged. The house is a white brick building with a jaunty pink and green trim. Zelma greets me at the door. We go into the television room, decorated in oranges and tans. Johnnie turns off the TV and greets me with a smile. He's wearing a plaid shirt and blue corduroy slacks. We exchange names and shake hands. He's an elderly man all right, with salt and pepper hair. His dark brown skin is so good, though, I can't guess how old he is. He's not wearing glasses, but I see a pair on the table next to him. And a quad cane nearby. He walks slowly back to his easy chair, sits down, and props his feet up. Zelma offers me a glass of water, which I gratefully accept. She sits to the side but pays close attention.

"How you doing?" he asks me.

"Real good, and yourself?"

"Not so bad . . . not so bad." Over the next hour he tells me his story, while Zelma adds her comments and reminders. Johnnie was a cook in the Army for seven years before opening his own fish business in St. Petersburg. "I married my bookkeeper," he says, nodding toward Zelma. She smiles.

"I was still working at eighty," he adds.

"And how old are you now?"

"I was born November 22, 1907," he says slowly. That would make him ninety-one at our interview. (Will I live that long? In such good health?)

We move on to his medical history. He speaks slowly and deliberately.

"Well, some years ago I had a stroke and my left leg went out. I basically had hypertension all along, but the symptoms got worse. I was confused but the stroke wasn't dramatic enough to get me to the doctor right away, so I waited a few days. When I went, he gave me aspirin. Things then went along pretty normal. We were never sure what that was.

"This Christmas I was sick again—kind of like a heart attack—but not a real classic MI. We went to the hospital. My heart was hardly putting out at all.

"I was frightened, I don't mind telling you. My family gathered around . . . and spoke with the cardiologist. They were over in a corner, but I could hear what they were saying. I guess I didn't have any real business listening, but I did anyway.

"My family doctor didn't think I'd come out of this at all and thought maybe we should put in a pacemaker. The cardiologist said no.

"Well, I was frightened, as I said, and asked the Lord to take care of me, my wife, and my daughter. It was just a little prayer, but I felt a lot better. I told the doctors to do what they needed to do. I figured whatever God's will was would be fine. It's the devil that's afraid. So they gave me a shot and I went to sleep. Then they did the cardioversion and I slept for about an hour. When I woke up, I felt fine."

The earlier stroke—if stroke it was—happened at home. Johnnie had some stroke-like events before that, possibly TIAs, transient ischemic attacks. In a

TIA, circulation in the brain is blocked for a small amount of time. The person may feel light-headed; fainting is possible.

In Johnnie's words, "I was a guard at a criminal complex when I passed out. I had rounds to make, you know, but I collapsed in a hallway and was unconscious for maybe an hour. When I woke up, I continued my rounds. I was generally weak and tired easily . . . short of breath. So we went to the doctor. I had an EKG, which showed an irregular heartbeat. They changed my medicines around. The cardiologist said I was doing as well as could be expected and that there didn't seem to be any permanent muscle damage to the heart. They sent me home on oxygen, and I had a home healthcare aide come for a while . . . for the bathing and such. I quit the oxygen myself. Too much bother for any benefit that I could tell. I would prop up in bed. And watch my diet. Zelma saw to that."

"Well," Zelma adds, "not too strictly. If you make it to these years, why worry too much? He likes ice cream, so I get him some of that. And I'll take a little bit too myself."

Johnnie continues, "My mother had hypertension . . . and died of it, so I've always been a little careful. No smoking, no drinking. They took my blood pressure when I went into the Army, and they said, 'Man, how in the world are you standing up?' Hell, I didn't know anything about it. Hypertension doesn't have any symptoms, you know. So they stuck me in the hospital and got me straightened around. A mighty good thing, too. I believe God takes care of us, often in strange ways. Reverend Terry and the church have been so good to me. He brings over communion now and then. That means a lot to me. He's sat with me when I was sick.

"But you can't give the Lord orders, you know, pray for specific things. You got to be patient. The Lord doesn't come when you call, but he's always on time." Johnnie smiles.

"I just take two medicines now, a pill for the hypertension and some aspirin. She makes up my tray," he says, nodding to Zelma. "Sometimes I try to skip something, but she raises hell if I do.

"I'm thankful, mostly. Being sick helps you sort things out. I used to think I needed a new car every year . . . now every three or four years is OK. You just don't need all the material things you think you do.

"So I pray, take the regular medicines, and we have other things too."
"Oh?"
"Shark cartilage, for one. Did you know sharks never get cancer?"

I nod out of politeness. I've read that sharks do, in fact, get cancer. Even if they didn't, what would be the mechanism to protect humans? Maybe it doesn't matter strictly speaking; the Reddicks seem to be getting the placebo benefit at least from such steps in taking responsibility to manage their health. The commercial exploitation of so-called "food additives" is, however, troubling to me. Americans spend billions of dollars a year on "dietary supplements" that may have no benefit or even cause outright harm (for example, interacting with prescribed medications).

Before I go, Zelma takes me into the formal living room to show me some angels she's made, figures about a foot high, all done up in white with haloes and wings. For me, their dark faces and hands contrast vividly with the white gowns, but I'm a white person who has seen mostly European images of angels. I'm touched that she would share these images with me, symbols of some of the deepest beliefs of this household. The word *angel*, I recall, means *messenger* in Greek. One sense of angels is a connection of our world with the world beyond, much like the portal of the Byzantine icon's eyes. If the Reddicks can feel protected and nourished by agents from the heavens, surely this must increase their sense of well-being and lower their stress. And, although I don't have the nerve to ask Johnnie about his sense of death, living with a group of angels and a loving wife surely must play some part in his understanding of this world and the next.

Valentines, Fencers, Cards: Cardiac Imagery

I remember making valentines in grade school. We'd carefully fold red construction paper in half then cut—with round-end scissors—from the folded edge to make a half a heart. I recall the delight of pulling the two sides apart to find a perfectly symmetrical heart opening itself to me. If the notch at the top wasn't deep enough, that could be touched up with another folded cut. I remember the resistance of the two layers of paper against my scissors. I remember the deeply saturated red of the paper. Sometimes we'd add a doily . . . remember the smell and cold feel of the paste? And then the questions arose. Who for? What to say? Parents and teachers were easy. Also good friends. But if there was some version of puppy love . . . or a crush . . . the difficulties of expression were immense. Language was difficult, the exact words impossible to find. The heart itself carried the message, a symbolic resonance of a tradition.

Images have a nonverbal power, or perhaps a super-verbal power, subsuming both the literal and figurative meanings of words. Zelma Reddick's angels, even her glass of water brought out to me, carried meanings of a host-guest relationship. In literature an image is an appeal to sense, such as taste or touch, but, especially, sight. Image is, of course, the root of the word *imagination*, the way we picture things and project desired realities.

Each year we school kids felt the excitement of preadolescent versions of love expressed with paper hearts, precursors to love letters of all sorts, and other gifts, such as gold locket hearts and gold heart earrings. While in graduate school I made a three-and-a-half-foot heart for a young woman whom I loved (and later married). As I carried it neatly folded in two across campus on a snowy February 14, I hoped it would be indiscernible, but other young women perceived its shape right away and smiled or outright giggled. Some images have immediate power, with stories suggested beyond them.

Besides valentines, there are heart images in this culture that tell us something about our desires. Red candy hearts, pastel conversation hearts, with messages of flirtation and affection printed on them. Red boxes of candy in heart shapes, cakes, hearts carved in tree bark, hearts drawn at the bottom of letters. All these and more tell us of the interest humans have in love, eros, and sex, and the symbolic power of the heart to represent them. Love and procreation are as central to the survival of our species as the biological heart is central to life. Romantic emotions cause the heart to beat faster . . . sexual activity causes the heart to beat faster. There' s a peak in pulse rate at orgasm and a blood pressure spike—evidence far removed from a delicate valentine of ribbons and doilies, but sometimes connected by a series of careful steps.

The shape of valentines is wonderfully appealing, whether in two or three dimensions. They vary, of course, with the cutter, drawer, or artisan—some taller, some thicker, but they almost always have the symmetry that suggests order, as opposed to the actual anatomical article, which is asymmetrical and blurred by the attachment of eight major blood vessels. The human heart has a taper (not a point) at the lower end, which is called an apex, and the upper margins are not notched like the valentine stylization. Many have noticed that the two upper swells of the valentine heart look like breasts or even the protuberant buttocks of, say, a woman bending over. Of the various face-shapes seen in women's magazines, the heart-shaped face is often called one of the more desirable—as if women could control this. In Julia Alvarez's wonderful novel, *How the García Girls Lost Their Accents* (Chapel Hill, N.C.: Algonquin Books, 1991), Yolanda has a heart-shaped face, with a widow's peak providing the upper, central accent.

The traditional red of valentines relates, of course, to blood, passion, eros, blushing, sex, flushes, and genital tumescence. The cupid's dart suggests that Dan Cupid has shot his arrow into the heart, wounding it and turning it inexorably toward love. The obvious Freudian reading would be the phallus entering the excited (red) and open (unfolded) female genitalia. More than one wag has suggested that the female pubic hair (medically styled as an "escutcheon," or shield) has a heart shape. In Günter Grass's novel *The Tin Drum* (1963), little Oskar is fascinated by his babysitter's patch and, somewhat confused, bites at it.

In *The Wizard of Oz* (1925), the Tin Man wants a heart. The rag dolls Raggedy Ann and Raggedy Andy have hearts sewn directly on their chests; children delight in showing these secret signs beneath the clothing. We sign letters with a ♥ to suggest the love that we are sending. Bumpers stickers abound with declarations of "I ♥ beagles/schnauzers/great danes," etc. Each of these provides a shorthand sign for love and affection and, more abstractly, for our own needs to receive such qualities. The manufacturer of one brand of heartworm pills provides little red hearts to apply to a calendar as a reminder for the monthly dose, as a symbol not only of the dog's biological heart but of the masters' love for their dogs, and the returned canine love. Children hope their dollies will love them; adults send love, hoping to receive it back.

Another heart icon with a different purpose is the traditional fencer's costume with a stylized red heart on the chest; here, of course, the meaning is not love, but physical vulnerability. This heart is usually somewhat misplaced, too high, too far to the side. When we say the Pledge of Allegiance with our hands over our hearts, often we put the hand in this higher, outer position. I imagine the symbolism is similar; we swear on our hearts, pledging our hearts and, therefore, our lives. Less dramatically, but more melodramatically, opera singers taking curtain calls make grand gestures to and from their hearts, suggesting their gratitude for applause (which they are also encouraging). A subtler version exists in Morocco: a fingertip tap on one's own sternum to indicate thanks.

According to Cirlot's *Dictionary of Symbols* (London: Routledge and K. Paul, 1971) the heart in medieval times was the image of the sun within humans, a hermetic version of gold, gold being the noble metal in alchemy. (Perhaps the modern version of alchemical transmutation from gross metals to gold is organ transplantation, including hearts, which can live a second time in another body.) The cliché of "the whore with a heart of gold" suggests a love beyond the merely carnal, pure and steadfast. A positive event "warms the cockles of the heart," the cockles being the deepest part of the heart. (A warm drink can do the same, owing to overlapping cardiac and gastric nerves.) Still, we interpret people and events according to our sense of their hearts (which may involve our sense of our own hearts).

In the world of playing cards, hearts are usually the second ranked suit, one below spades. The four traditional suits originated in Italy, representing four classes of society from the highest to the lowest: spades meant swords or the military, hearts stood for the church, while diamonds stood for tradespeople, and clubs were for husbandmen and peasants. (The card game of Hearts is a rare instance of hearts being considered negative; players try to avoid taking these cards.)

The largest single image of a human heart that I've encountered is the "Giant Heart" at the Franklin Institute in Philadelphia. This multicolored heart is about the size of two school buses combined, so that the heart model is scaled up some forty times from normal human size. It's as if the designers had read the quotation cited earlier about a child crawling through a whale's heart and decided to go one better. Surrounded by hordes of children who yelled and jumped and shrieked throughout this cardiac fun house, I walked and climbed through it three times; the Giant Heart has steps and walkways tall enough for an adult to walk upright, all the while hearing *LUB DUB* at 72 beats a minute and, during the passage near the lungs, a rhythmic squishing sound. At this point images of blood vessels projected on the floor turn from blue to red, to suggest their uptake of oxygen. Signs announce the structures of chambers, valves, and blood vessels; some children read these, but more, in my brief observation, did not. What they experienced, I think, was a more intuitive lesson of the spatial flow within the heart, intensified by the multisensory impressions of sight, sound, and touch. As they hollered and careened around the pathways curving up and down, they got a visceral sense of the intricate genius of the organ, a sense that I hope stays with them at one level of consciousness or another. The Giant Heart is the centerpiece of a huge room—some five thousand square feet—dedicated to the heart. Another eighteen exhibits include hearts of various sizes from animals, an open-heart operation with a dummy whose chest is a TV screen showing the surgery, and a dynamic blood volume demonstration. A person stands on a scale and red liquid pours into a column to show ten, twenty, or thirty pints, corresponding to that person's weight. Young men boasted about how much blood they had and jockeyed for the chance to display their liquid vitality. Throughout this large room children excitedly participated in one exhibit after another, their imaginations energized by the clever displays. It seemed to me that this city of brotherly love offered here an experience of *philakardia*, or heart love, both in the sense that the room was a celebration of hearts and that the pervasive health messages urged us to love our hearts and, therefore, to take care of them.

One day at my ER in Florida, a man comes in by helicopter, a pedestrian hit by a car. "Ped vs. car" is the cryptic note on the white board that hangs on the door of Trauma 2. "Ped" or "Bike" versus a car is usually bad news for the patient. This man is, indeed, seriously injured and cannot talk, so Doug, one of the chaplains, and I must go through his wallet to figure out his identity and therefore whom to call. We don't find any driver's license, insurance card, or other evidence of home or relatives. The police on the case say that he's a street person but that he does have a job. Doug finds a card for his employer and leaves to make that call. In closing the wallet, I take another look at the very first card we saw. It's a picture of Jesus in bright colors, with a large heart—larger than an ordinary human heart—drawn on his chest, a symmetrical valentine heart centered on the midline. Bursts of light extend from it in all directions. A crown of thorns surrounds it at the widest part. A cross floats above it. On the back of the card I read, "Learn of me, for I am meek and humble of heart (Mt. 11.29)." Where many of us might keep a driver's license—our symbol of power, citizenship, identity—this man places this symbolic image, the first thing he sees whenever he opens his wallet. Perhaps it works apotropaically for him, warding off evil; or perhaps it is a talisman, a blessing.

In Catholic tradition, the Sacred Heart of Jesus, whether drawn, painted, or sculpted, suggests his enormous capacity for love, especially in the energetic bursts of light, a variation on an aura or halo. Specifically, Margaret Mary Alacoque, a French nun, had reported a revelation in 1677, in which Jesus, fresh from scourging, revealed his Sacred Heart to her and made twelve promises that he would fulfill to persons who practiced devotion to this heart. She wrote in a letter, "The sacred heart of Christ is an inexhaustible fountain and its sole desire is to pour itself out into the hearts of the humble so as to free them and prepare them to lead lives according to his good pleasure." Graphically, this spiritual projection has power and universality: its rays extend in all directions, available to all persons. The heart itself suggests a purer love than the erotic, a sacrificial love symbolized by the crown of thorns and, of course, the cross.

There's also a Sacred Heart of Mary, the scriptural source for which is Luke 2.19 ("And Mary kept all these things and pondered them in her heart"); thus her heart combines her love for her newborn son (as well as for all other persons) with her wisdom in weighing truth, attributes suitable for an intercessory figure between humans and the divine. As many (including William Butler Yeats) have pointed out, the classic Christian trinity of Father, Son, and Holy Spirit is typically considered totally male, but the addition of Mary gives a female dimension, a female "heartedness." (In earlier Hebrew tradition, the Hagia Sophia—or Holy Spirit—was originally female, an intuitive wisdom that was overwhelmed later by masculine rationalism.) Numerous Catholic churches, schools, colleges, and universities are called Sacred Heart, including the highly visible Sacre Coeur in Paris.

For our injured street person, a man without a home, the Sacred Heart of Jesus was an image that provided an abode of protection and love.

Religion and the Heart

Many religious traditions have used the heart as a symbol, although the word "symbol" doesn't seem dynamic enough—in contrast with the icon we saw earlier. Furthermore, some heart symbols are large, even epic in scope, suggesting links between the natural and the supernatural world. The ancient Egyptians chose the weighing of soul—concretized as the heart—to show the worth of a person's life at death. I have seen a papyrus depicting this scene in the British Museum: Anubis weighs the heart on a large balance, the heart on one side, a feather on the other, while Thoth and the monster Amenait watch. The feather symbolizes the goddess Maat, or truth. If the heart is deemed guilty, Ammit—part lion, part hippopotamus, part crocodile—devours the heart. If the heart balances, the soul moves on to the kingdom of Osiris, the afterworld. As the mummy is wrapped up, the heart was the only organ of the viscera left in the body, an indispensable soul-center. Even the brain was drained out of the nose with a long wire and discarded.

According to James Morris, the word "heart" appears some 132 times in the Qur'an, meaning the physical heart only two or three times. Instead, heart here means a meeting place of God and human, an influence of divine intentions upon our wills and, therefore, our actions, even to the point of God's responsibility within us. A Sufi saying puts it this way: "The heart of the person of faith is the Throne of the All-Merciful."

In the Hindu traditions of yoga, the heart chakra (or *anahata*) is very important, the center of spiritual or divine love. As we saw earlier, chakras are energy wheels aligned along the spine, through which energy passes. Stephen Sturgess's *The Yoga Book* (Rockport, Mass.: Element, 1997) shows that each yogic chakra corresponds to an endocrine gland and a nerve plexus, the structures identified by western medicine. The heart chakra corresponds to the thymus and, of course, to the cardiac plexus. Caroline Myss extends such correspondences in her book *Anatomy of the Spirit: The Seven Stages of Power and Healing* (New York: Three Rivers Press, 1996). For her, the Hindu chakras, the Christian sacraments, and the Jewish Kabbalah overlap different cultural interpretations of the human body, mind, and spirit, including, of course, the heart. In her chapter on the fourth chakra, the center of the chest, she writes, "Healing begins with the repair of emotional injuries. Our entire medical model is being reshaped around the power of the heart." Further, she finds, the heart energy and the head energy need to be in balance. In general, Myss sees emotional health and physical health intertwined, especially through body energy.

In the Mahayana Buddhist tradition, the "Prajnaparamita Heart Sutra" is a central document; "Just as we hold the heart to be the center, that sutra holds the essence of all the Prajnaparamita texts," explains Grand Master T'an Hsu. Gretel Ehrlich wrote in *A Match to the Heart* that she found comfort in this sutra after she was struck by lightning; the main message of the sutra is rather abstract, however, not using the human heart in any incarnated way.

In some American Indian traditions, the heartline is an arrow representing the pathway of breath from an animal's head to its heart, showing its life force of animal spirit. The heartline is drawn or carved on the side of an animal, from its snout or front of its chest to its midchest. The International Heart Institute of Montana uses a horse with such a line as its emblem. Zuni fetishes (small animals, typically carved in stone) have a heartline inscribed; for this culture, these fetishes have magical powers.

Religious uses of heart imagery tend to emphasize center or essence, wisdom (or true knowledge), courage, and generosity, reminiscent of meanings we found earlier in discussing heart phrases. Religions tend not to use the more secular, more earthy meanings, however, such as passion, emotions, the erotic. On the other hand, religious uses expand our sense of heart to the holy, the numinous, the spiritual, the beyond—realms we don't talk about much in modern secular culture; without a common language for religion, we either have no tradition or a personal, particular faith that we rarely discuss with outsiders. And the body—especially in the mass media—has become largely erotically charged, another level of consciousness from the reverence Michael Curry spoke of that still pertains, at least for some, to the heart.

Young's *Analytical Concordance of the Bible* lists that the word "heart" occurs in the Old Testament over eight hundred times (i.e., the Hebrew Bible) and the New Testament. The Hebrew is *leb,* and the Greek, *kardia.* In the Noah story, we find that God regrets creating man, "and it grieved him in his heart," because man's "imagination of the thoughts of his heart was only evil" (Genesis 6:5–6). Pharaoh "hardens his heart" against the Hebrews (Exodus 7:13, 14, etc.). Heart, according to the editors of the Oxford Annotated Bible, typically means "mind" and "will," including ways these are expressed in action. This notion is well illustrated in the Shema (Deuteronomy 6:4–9), a classic statement of faith, and in Deuteronomy 6:13–22. (These two passages are contained in the mezuzah, a small container attached to the doorframe of a house, a sign of faith for Jewish households.) Moses is speaking in the two passages, part of his second address to his people. The Shema begins, "Hear, O Israel: The LORD our God is one LORD; and you shall love the LORD with all your heart, and with all your soul, and with all your might. And these words which I command you this day shall be upon your heart" (Revised Standard Version). Given that Moses is describing the terms of the covenant between God and Israel, we can see that the heart is a place of commitment, resolve, and connection with God. Moses urges his people, in a bold image, to "Circumcise therefore the foreskin of your heart, and be no longer stubborn" (Deuteronomy 10:16). Just as the circumcision of the penis marks the men of Israel as descendants of Abraham, as God's chosen tribe, the inner person should also be marked as a servant of God.

Conscience, sense of probity, even guilt also can reside in heart, as seen in David's story (1, 2 Samuel); twice we read that David's "heart smote him" in his duties as king—although oddly enough not after his seduction of Bathsheba. The Psalms (traditionally said to be written in part by David) are rich with heart references, some 159, averaging more than one per psalm. Here the heart symbolizes inner wisdom, the quality of will, resolve, and conscience: "He who has clean hands and a pure heart" (24), "the strength of my heart" (72), "My heart is ready, O God" (108). One of the most famous passages, often set to music, begins "Create in me a clean heart, O God" (51), suggesting that the heart is a meeting place for God's love and power and human desire to act justly, despite propensities for sin. Similarly, the Old Testament prophets call for the return of hearts to God—stubborn hearts, proud hearts, false hearts—and the failure to lay knowledge of God "to your hearts." Again, the heart symbolizes the inner nature of persons (and tribes) and a place where humans and God can meet. In a tenor aria in Mendelssohn's oratorio *Elijah*, Obadiah exhorts the tribe, "'If with all your hearts you truly seek me, ye shall ever surely find me,' thus saith our God."

In Proverbs 17:22, we find an early realization of connections between mind and body: "A cheerful heart is a good medicine, but a downcast spirit dries up the bones." Ecclesiastes 9:7 exhorts, "drink your wine with a merry heart." And the lovers of Song of Solomon sing, "Set me as a seal upon your heart," a symbolic mark of intimate union; the seal is a sign of ownership and authority, as in a king's seal upon a letter, or, again, the Hebraic circumcision. If the passage is read at a spiritual level, it could be the tribe of Israel calling for God's ownership and protection.

In the New Testament, the same imagery and themes continue. Jesus himself quotes the first portion of the Shema in answer to what is the greatest commandment (Mark 12:29–30). In his Beatitudes (Matthew 5:3–12) Jesus says, "Blessed are the pure in heart," and he also warns that a person should not commit "adultery in his heart" (Matthew 5:27), stressing the importance of the inner life and quality of our thoughts. Four times Jesus urges people to "take heart," usually as he heals them. As we saw earlier, Mary, thinking about the birth of Jesus and the visitation of the shepherds, "kept all these things and pondered them in her heart" (Luke 2:19), a more reflective, introspective version of the heart. In his Epistles, Paul urges us to "singleness of heart" and a "pure heart." And in Revelations, the risen Lord proclaims, "I am he who searches mind and heart, and I will give to each of you as your works deserve" (Revelations 2:23).

Heart imagery in the Bible is varied in its themes, but fairly consistent in emphasizing the human qualities of will, mind, resolve, and conscience, as well as essential moral nature. One Hebrew and English lexicon of the Old Testament translates *leb* not only as "heart," but as "inner man, mind, will, moral character, the seat of appetites, reflection, memory," and "seat of courage," amply showing the wide range of possible meanings and levels of human excellence. Humans can be noble in their hearts or follow desire or even sin; they can harden their hearts, or they can implore God to create within them new hearts, but God always seeks a meeting place in the heart. Renaissance poet John Donne continues this tradition in his dramatic Holy Sonnet 14 when he cries, "Batter my heart, three-personed God," calling for God to attack and subdue his sinful heart.

Scholar Olivia McIntyre has traced some of the medieval iconography of the heart; in art, it represents love, piety, and charity. Anointing with oil on the breast symbolizes purifying the heart, allowing God to instill his spirit in human beings. The heart was a symbol for two Sienese saints, and, more rarely, St. Augustine. Considering the heart as spiritually separate from the body and perfectible helps explain the burial of hearts of French royalty separate from their bodies. While their bodies—the royal embodiment of the public kingship—all went to St. Denys, the heart—the private, personal, and spiritual aspect—could be buried wherever the king chose, often a place of special holiness. And not only kings: some church officials and nobility had their hearts buried at a church in Paris cared for by Celestine monks. McIntyre writes, "Perhaps the most colorful example of heart-burial comes from Scottish history with Robert Bruce's ill-fated attempt to have his heart buried in the Church of the Holy Sepulchre in Jerusalem."

Nowadays, we usually see our hearts as active pumps or organs needing medical attention, not places of purity, conscience—let alone meeting places with the divine. The one common request for a different burial place is implied in the gift of heart transplantation: the donor goes to the grave without his or her heart, and the transplanted organ—if successful—is in a person unknown, a person whose future death is unforeseeable in place or in time. In Richard Selzer's short story "Whither Thou Goest," a woman pursues a man who is the recipient of her husband's heart until she can hear it beating, once again, in the new location.

GEORGE'S GUT PERFORATES, IS PRAYED OVER

On Wednesday afternoons, I go the emergency room to visit patients.

"Hi, my name's Howard. I'm a volunteer from the Chaplain's office." We shake hands.

"How are you feeling?" I ask. Some patients look my green jacket over, reading my name from my badge and the words "Pastoral Care." Some will say, "Does this mean I'm dying," either as a joke or as an actual fear. A few wonder whether I'll proselytize. (I don't.) Some are particularly glad to see someone religious and ask if I'm a minister. "No, I'm a layperson," I explain. Almost all are glad to have someone to talk to, especially someone nonmedical; ER patients are usually afraid, lonely, and/or bored. My job is to listen, to make phone calls, and to help give voice to unspoken concerns. A tough guy sketches details of his accident. "Sounds scary," I say. "You're damn right," he says.

As a 501(c)(3)—hospital (according to the tax code provision), we are obligated to receive any patient who shows up at our doors. Some of these will never pay a nickel, even though the basic charge for the ER starts at about ninety dollars. Street people, for example, never pay, and the hospital gives away such care ("eats the bill"). Others, with no regular doctor, use us as a clinic. This is inefficient and inappropriate, of course, but evidently the best the U.S. health-care "system" can currently provide. Clearly every one, rich or poor, becomes sick or is injured sooner or later, as time and chance happen to us all. (Or maybe this is not so clear to America as a whole, given that we don't have a national health care system that can protect, especially, children, the aged, the poor.) At my ER I've met ocean-going sailors from the harbor nearby. I've met tourists from all the inhabited continents. I've met people who have attempted suicide, a five-hundred-pound man (who needed a heavy-duty stretcher), a woman 108 years old, and a 3-year-old boy with beautiful blue eyes, comatose from a near drowning. I've talked with people struck by lightning, a woman who assured me that she was from another planet, a man who survived his jump off the Sunshine Skyway, falling two hundred feet to the water. Besides the unusual people, we have the usual range of car wrecks, home and work accidents, falls, asthma attacks, heart attacks, diabetic crises, muggings, suicide attempts—and everything else. Whether the illness or accident is bizarre or commonplace, patients are suddenly bumped out of their daily routine. Some are angry; some are sad; some are afraid; most feel loneliness as they lie isolated in their beds. Some, when faced with their mortality, wonder about their souls: as the proverb has it, "There are no atheists in fox holes." Religious persons are often immediately glad to see me, elderly African-Americans, in particular. When I asked one women how she felt, she said, "I'm so thankful. I'm very thankful. My body's falling apart, but I'm *thankful*." She understood being healthy in the midst of unhealth.

Wednesday afternoon is my volunteering time at the hospital. I go to the office to sign in; I riffle through the card file. When I get to my card I'm surprised to find a note paper clipped to it. What the heck? I unfold it and find a message from my minister: *George is undergoing emergency abdominal surgery, possibly for a perforated bowel.* Damn! George Meese is a fellow professor; he's one of my best friends. I hasten up to the OR area. Since my green volunteer's jacket can get me in almost anywhere, I enter the OR suite and ask the charge nurse about George.

"They're just coming out now," she says. Sure enough, a Rube Goldberg-style gurney carries George in a cloth sling. He looks pale.

"What's the deal?" I ask a nurse.

"He perfed. We fixed him up."

I go on down to my usual stint in the emergency room, knowing he won't be waking up in post-op for some time. Later in the day I visit his room.

"George?" I say. He's on his back in bed. His midsection is heavily bandaged.

"Oh, Howard . . . they thought they might have to take the colon out and rip me a new one. You know, I'd be on a bag . . ." his voice trails off.

Two days later a group of six of us from our church come for a laying on of hands. We enter the room and surround the bed. Since George, an elder at the church, knows everyone, there are no introductions. Nor small talk either. We put our hands on him from both sides and from the foot of the bed. Elder Nancy Appunn gives a prayer:

"Holy God, it's a beautiful day outside, with sun, with breezes, with the song of birds. But your servant George lies here, sick, afraid, and separated from those he loves. We ask your blessing on George today and call for your healing presence to be with him. Heal his surgery and calm his mind. We know that long hours in bed can be a time of loneliness and worry. Companion him here and free him from anxious cares so that this be a time of rest and healing for him. Let George know that we love him now and in the hours to come, regardless of the distance between us. We ask it in Jesus's name. Amen."

The rest of us say, "Amen" and we all file out.

I find the ceremony powerful. What did George feel?

I find out the next day. George is sitting up in bed. He looks pinker, more alert. I don't have time to ask about the laying on of hands . . . he's telling me already.

"It was so funny yesterday when the nurse came after you guys visited. She took my vital signs twice, thinking she was making mistakes. Then she grabbed the chart and said, 'Did you get some meds I don't know about? Your pulse is down, your BP is way down, your respirations are down.' I told her people from my church came and prayed over me. I left it up to her to decide what happened in my body, but just watching her puzzlement made me feel good."

"I would have liked to have seen that."

"Yeah, but the main thing is the power of prayer with people you trust. And it's had a lasting effect too. I'm going to get out of here sooner than they were thinking, it looks like."

Later, George shared some writing about the event:

In an operation like this there is a very critical time when the body is either going to work again or not. The difference is a prospective life of normal length and reasonable ability, or a life of about six to ten years of constant disability and an early death; in worst-case situations, even death within a week. The doctors hadn't told me all of that—just that I should be "functioning" within two days—and that was then more than a day ago. Besides the pain of being cut across the abdomen from hipbone to hipbone, I was becoming very worried, fearful, and even panicked that I was not responding—that my body was going to shut down.

And after our laying on of hands and prayer:

Almost immediately, the most profound peace I have ever felt poured over me—the sensation was almost water-like—a perceptible "flowing" of calming confidence in, or union with, something much, much larger than everyone in that room, that hospital, this city. My panic evaporated. Within an hour, my vital signs perked up, the operation proved successful, and I began healing in ways I had never imagined.

What happened? Let's say there are two groups of possible explanations.

Group A includes the following. As trusted people provided this ritual to George, he felt a sense of solidarity, a sense that he was loved and cared for. Once again he felt that he was as human as his visitors, as the touch of our hands, at twelve places over his body, reconnected him not only with his colleagues but with his own body, which we were not afraid to touch. The words of the prayer captured his sense of isolation, his fears, and his immediate urges to return to work and to dispel all of these. Reconnected with persons and a shared sense of the supernatural, he felt contexted, even in his bed and bandages.

Group B is short: God answered the prayer with a miracle.

Or is there a Group C? What if the group A explanations—the more secular, rational reading of the event—may be understood as ways God works, spirit incarnated in the words and hands of fellow humans?

A few years later I hear Dr. Herbert Benson speak. He's the author of *The Relaxation Response* (New York: Avon, 1975) and a leader in finding ways mind and body can work together in healing. Benson, ordinarily at Harvard, was speaking in St. Petersburg. He said that men recovering from heart surgery who belong to some significant community have a 50 percent lower morbidity rate than men who don't. If that significant community is a worshiping religious community, the morbidity rate drops to 90 percent. Other research seems to support the influences of religious belief upon health care. The National Institute for Healthcare Research (not a governmental organization but supported by the John Templeton Foundation) surveys current medical and sociological literature and reports findings. Some of the articles in recent years show that patients' spirituality is linked to better overall health (*Family Medicine*, 1998); that attending church is linked with lower blood pressure, lower deaths from cardiovascular disease, and, more generally, living longer (*American Journal of Public Health*, 1998); that religious service attendance correlates with social support networks, both of which are health-promoting (*Journal of the Scientific Study of Religion*, 1995); that persons with an active religious faith recover better from heart transplant surgery, feeling less anxiety and higher self-esteem (*Journal of Religion and Health*, 1995); and that elderly heart patients are fourteen times less likely to die following surgery if they are both socially active and have religious faith (*Psychosomatic Medicine*, 1995). A review of seventy-eight different studies found that religion significantly enhances physical health, along with five other contributing factors: lifestyle choices, social support, hope, comfort, and positive effects of prayer (*Journal of Psychology and Christianity*, 1995).

Larry Dossey has written about prayer and health. When I heard him speak in 1996, he said he was initially skeptical about influences of religion on health and that he believed his research would disprove any links. In the course of researching his book *Healing Words: The Power of Prayer and the Practice of Medicine* (San Francisco: Harper San Francisco, 1993), however, he changed his mind. Dossey reviewed over a hundred studies and considered his own experience as a physician, concluding that "at least some of the time, *it* [prayer] *works.*" He also sees a larger picture: "It is now possible to tell a new story, one that allows science and spirituality to stand side by side in a complementary way, neither trying to usurp or eliminate the other." More specifically, Dossey favors generic prayers ("Thy will be done"; "May the best possible outcome prevail") over specific requests, and he emphasizes "a sense of empathy or emotional closeness"—which he calls "a heart connection" between well people and sick people, physicians and patients, even humans and animals. Dossey's work has been controversial within the medical community; indeed Stephen Barrett's Quackwatch Web site calls *Healing Words* "nonrecommended." There is, however, a trend that doctors understand religious belief as an ally for patients and, often, for themselves. Roughly half of U.S. medical schools now teach students to ask questions about religious belief as part of the social history of a patient.

While the end of the twentieth century found extraordinary developments in surgical and medical cardiology, the beginning of the twenty-first century may find other, complementary ways to heal the human heart. Not only because medical science may be evolving that way, but also because a majority of patients will be asking for such support. Religion and health polls (CBS, *USA Weekend, Time*) agree that about 80 percent of Americans believe that spiritual faith or prayer can help people recover from disease, and about two-thirds believe that doctor and patient should talk about religious matters.

I Go to the Hospital with Crushing Chest Pain

It's Sunday morning, and I'm talking with my friend Bruce between church services. It's a lovely day in St. Petersburg, and we're sipping orange juice. Worship in the first service was satisfying, and my choir sang well. I'm feeling good about my life in general, but my chest is suddenly tight. I think it might be stomach or bowel distress and go to the bathroom . . . with no relief. I find my wife and tell her I don't feel well. The pain increases minute to minute. I think, *this could be a lot of things, but heart attack is one very good possibility.* I sit down on a bench. People look at me, alarmed. One says, "You look white." My strength is flowing out of me. I feel totally helpless. I ask my wife to drive me to the emergency room. She brings the car nearby and Bruce and Walt help me to it, one supporting each of my arms. On our ten-minute drive, my breath comes shorter, and I start to sweat. My forearms and hands tingle. *Is this the big one?* As much as I believe in primary research . . . the irony of my having a heart attack while writing on hearts is surely too much! The pain is overwhelming. It feels as though a torturer is tightening a band around me or—as many have said—I'm being crushed by an elephant.

Nancy drives me to the ambulance entrance, making my family three for three at this ER: daughter/collarbone, wife/ruptured appendix, me/Something Bad. This is where I volunteer, so I know a lot of folks. They'd give anyone good service, of course, and quickly, especially if the admitting complaint is what I gasp out to the clerk: "Possible MI."

"Take off your shirt," says Anne, tall and regal, one of my favorite nurses. She leads me to CCA, a small room for acute care. Chris (one of my students!) applies the EKG leads. Someone else puts a Hep Lock in the back of my hand for IV access. The pain in my chest is unrelenting, like nothing I've ever felt. It's a dull area about the size of two open hands around and below my right nipple. I can barely talk. Nurses and docs ask if it radiates to the back (no) or down my left arm (no), classic signs for an MI. I'm scared, of course, and my first BP is 143/90, way high for me. The first drug in the IV barely touches my pain, but the second erases it like magic. It's a narcotic that puts me on cloud nine, although I'm still conscious and coherent. I mention this to Beth, a Peds nurse who drops by, and she says with a smile, "Now you know what illegal drugs are all about." My wife is there, my choir director Mike, my fellow singer Carolyn, and one of my ministers, Holly. I'm grateful for their support and care. I run the chant in my mind, "Thy will be done, thy will be done," and try to breathe deeply.

Dr. Lozano gives me the initial report: the EKG looks good, and cardiac enzymes are OK, but these may not change immediately if there's been damage to the heart. He says heart and gallbladder are the two leading candidates. Do I want the double doors to my treatment room closed and the curtains drawn? Of course not . . . I'm an extrovert. Various nurses, the unit clerk stop by; they usually see me active in my green volunteer's jacket. Now I'm in my hospital gown trying to get comfortable on the hard bed. I ask them about gallbladders and learn that gallstones, even "sludge," can block the outflow duct and cause considerable pain. I'm wheeled down to Ultrasound to check out my chest, the gallbladder in particular. The technician says she sees no stones. I'm disappointed, since that suggests heart again. My narcotic helps me nap the rest of the afternoon away, despite hustle and bustle around me; my bed's been rolled out into the hall. Someone needs CCA worse than I do. I recall that one of my students died in that room some years ago; I was sent down the hall to get blood for her.

The next day Dr. Carlson from my family practice group comes to my hospital room. I'm on the fourth floor, the cardiac floor, where I have volunteered; indeed, I've visited patients in this very room. Now it's me in bed with a hospital gown. In a pocket over my sternum is a gray plastic box, the radio relay for a continuous EKG. Antennas in the hall listen to me and the other patients all day and night and send the information to monitors at the nursing station.

"Well, with the heart, and someone your age," Dr. Carlson says, "we need to be very careful, very conservative." My age . . . fifty-six—closer to the edge! Every day in the obituaries I see ages within five years of mine.

He continues, "The ultrasound didn't show anything in the gallbladder, so we still have to think heart. On the other hand, the repeated cardiac enzymes and EKGs look normal. This is suggestive and encouraging, but not definitive. We'll try a HIDA test for the gallbladder. If that's positive, we'll know what direction to go, since the likelihood of your having both gallbladder *and* heart is virtually nil."

My roommate is an elderly man, Trent. He looks about eighty, but the nurse reads sixty-one off his chart. He coughs a lot. Since he cannot speak; our communication is limited. He sleeps most of the time. I say a prayer for him. When I was a pastoral care volunteer on this floor, I'd start in the cardiac intensive care unit and see patients in their glass cubicles. Most were unresponsive, given their illness and/or drugs. Then I'd move to the floor, including the room I'm in now. These patients were usually stable and most were eager to leave. Many had plenty of visitors, making me unnecessary. It was easy to see who was going home soon; I remember one vital, tanned woman who was anxious to get back to playing tennis.

In the morning I wonder whether to bother shaving . . . or should I lapse into passivity? No, I decide, and I shave and change my gown. I walk around in the halls. I visit the nurses' station and watch the purple line of my EKG march across a monitor. There were six other lines in different colors. One nurse says, "Yours looks fine. But look at this poor guy here," pointing to a yellow line, all uneven and jagged.

Doug Harrell, one of the hospital chaplains, comes to see me. I usually see him in the emergency room during trauma alerts. Sandy Giles, the parish nurse from my church, brings me a chocolate milkshake made with yogurt. All three of us hold hands while Doug prays out loud—much as Nancy Appunn did for George—and we include Trent in the next bed. Such visits and various phone calls mean a lot to me; they help hold me in the world of the healthy, even while I'm living in the world of the sick.

At noon—without breakfast (or lunch, it turns out)—I get wheeled down to the nukes lab, a place much like the Missoula lab described in "Looking into the Heart" in Michael's section. Technician Kelley injects a technetium-marked drug into my IV; it collects in the gallbladder, but doesn't leak down the bile duct like it should—according to the machine I'm lying under. She tells me to walk around to see if anything will shake loose. I walk. I shake. I jump up and down. Then another technician, Jose, has me lie down under another induction head (or camera) and injects another drug into my IV. This one is an enzyme that might unclog me. He points to a black and white monitor above me with a fuzzy image like a thumb print. "That's your gallbladder. We want to see a tail growing out of it. And over there," he gestures to a color monitor, "are the gradients." Sure enough, the liver is a series of purple dots scattered over most of the screen—it didn't uptake much of the radiopharmaceutical. But the gallbladder is precise and vivid in glorious red, an aggressive strawberry, with a thin border of orange. When Kelley stops by I ask her if I can do anything to move the bile, perhaps through my breathing. She says no, but encourages me to think of fatty foods—steak, potatoes with butter, lobster, since bile helps digest fats in the small intestine. I try varieties of breathing anyway and also create in my mind lavish, piggish meals. First, bacon and eggs, dripping with fat, then a greasy lunch of hamburgers, fries, a spoonful of lard for dessert, and a dinner of all she suggested plus a mammoth hot fudge sundae. I watch the two monitors and see bile leaking downward—in white, in blue—and into the small intestine in an ess shape. I'm thrilled. I'm saved! My eyes tear up. Jose says, however, that we need to get an ejection fraction of 48 percent within thirty minutes for the bladder to be considered normal. At the end of the test, my gallbladder has diminished some, but not the magical 48 percent. In sum, it will probably be interpreted as abnormal. I may need surgery. But it isn't my heart, and I'm grateful for that.

What did I learn? Total, debilitating pain totally changes how you live in the world, even which world you feel you live in: severe chest pain cuts you off from the ordinary, normal world of the well. The pain, stress, and worry—all reinforced by the unfamiliar trappings and routines of a hospital—put you in the world of the sick or even dying. Phone calls, visits, a card, a prayer can give you quite a lift, well out of proportion to how small they may seem to the giver. Such signs from the outside world of the well help reconnect you to that world, to recontext you, even if only temporarily, to the world of the healthy and out of the world of the sick. I also found that good doctors, nurses, technicians, and clerks are worth their weight in gold. Finally, I had the sense that there is an art to being a patient, to letting go, to trusting in whatever outcome, but at the same time not becoming totally passive.

Returning to the world of the well is a joyous experience, and it's easy to forget the pain and separation of the hospital. It's easy to fall right back into the busy routines of the "normal" world and to forget about sick people, those who care for them, and the mortality we all share.

The following Wednesday I go back to the ER, this time vertical and in my green jacket. I thank some of the people who took care of me and explain about the gallbladder. It's busy today; most beds are full. We have two traumas, and a code who does not survive, although drugs keep his heart going for a while. I talk with a dozen patients, including a man named Dylan, who lies in the bed in CCA, where I was three days before. He has white, thinning hair, and his skin is good. I can't tell how old he is. When I ask, he says, "Guess." I try sixty and he just laughs. His Jamaican accent has faded with time, but his sense of values has not. He tells me that he grew up with fifteen brothers and sisters, all of whom became educated and got good jobs.

"It's not hard. My parents had nothing, but we all pitched in. If someone needed good shoes for something, we lent them one of the few pairs. You need faith and good effort; the Lord will take care of everything else."

I ask how he feels. He clearly has a wicked cough and a fever.

"Oh, I feel fine. I'm sick today, but I've been sick before. I had five heart attacks in seven years when I was in business. Some people are slow on the uptake, but I finally saw the light and got out of business. I joined a Catholic community. I've raised eight adopted daughters. It's not hard. You have to see things in terms of *yes*. Most people see things in terms of *no*."

"Yeah . . . I had a minister named Lacy Harwell who would often include in his benediction, 'Live your hopes and not your fears.'"

"That's it," Dylan smiled. "It's not hard. It's not hard at all."

TAKING FOOD TO HEART

"Heart Smart Dinner" the notice read on the church bulletin board. An evening program: come at 6:00 to eat, 6:30 for just the program. Should I go? Certainly we've all heard about cholesterol and the steaks and butter we shouldn't eat so as to keep our arteries healthy. But there's probably more to the picture than that. This series of programs at our church is, in fact, new. We have a parish nurse, an energetic woman named Sandy Giles, a registered nurse on loan to us through a grant for one year. A parish nurse—what a great idea. We have many older people in our church. In our services, we pray for persons with cancer, persons who have fallen, persons who are dying or recently dead, and the like. A church is a life-span organization; for better or worse, all younger people can see possibilities of illness, disability, and death that lie in their future. And we can all consider what stewardship we might take over our bodies.

My wife had emergency surgery for a burst appendix the previous spring, not long after our return from Montana. Instead of the usual two-day hospital stay, she was there for six days with IV antibiotics sluicing through her to clean up some peritonitis. In any other century, she'd be dead. Since current practice is not to close the skin, she had a four-inch wound left wide open, with the subdermal fat visible. "You're not squeamish, are you," her nurse at the hospital said to me, since I'd be doing the dressing changes.

"Not much," said I, "but I thought she'd have nice neat stitches like railroad tracks."

"We used to do that, but we have fewer abscesses this way. She can take this wound right into the shower and put soap right on it." *What?* I thought. For reassurance, I called up our new parish nurse and explained the situation.

"How deep is the wound?" Sandy asked.

"A half inch at the deepest."

"Oh, that's nothing. I've seen them four inches deep, and still they heal up. We call it healing by primary intention—the body knows what to do. She'll do fine."

My mind eased, I changed the dressings as required and passed along the comforting information to Nancy—who healed routinely. Care for body and soul isn't that what the church should be about?—despite the puritanical strain that pretends that we have no bodies at all. I've heard of churches that have gyms, even swimming pools. If the body is a temple for the soul as the apostle Paul said, shouldn't we keep it in good shape for worship?

At 6:00 P.M. I park at the church and enter the narthex, where two women are setting up to serve our supper. I want to peek under the big stainless steel covers because something smells good. I walk to the multipurpose room where the talk will be. I see, predictably, several white heads. Older folks like events like this; they like the fellowship, regardless of topic, but they're also concerned about their health, and some are, specifically, heart patients. There's one glaring exception: a thirtyish blonde who sits by herself . . . probably tonight's speaker. I take the last empty seat at a table for six; my dining companions are at a minimum one decade older than me. Two are widows. Did their husbands die of heart disease? In the course of our small talk, Estelle, across the table from me, mentions that she was married for sixty-three years.

"You must have been a child bride," I gallantly offer.

"Not me. I married at twenty-five. I'm an old woman now," she says matter-of-factly. How refreshing, I think; how wonderful: someone comfortable with being old. I look at her wrinkles, her old-timey rings, her merry blue eyes. This seems to be a person who followed Socrates' injunction: *know thyself.*

Sandy, in her nurse's white jacket, offers a prayer and describes the food. "The chicken breasts are stuffed with herbs and baked. There's salad, mixed vegetables—steamed, naturally—and bread. Butter is available for those who are addicted." She laughs. "Dessert is cake with fruit ladled over." Of course: low-fat, healthy stuff. The six tables empty out, and we line up to load our plates. The food is attractively displayed and inviting—a certifiably healthy meal. As we eat, we say how good it tastes. I find myself eating more slowly, savoring each bite. How could you measure the health benefits of satisfaction and good company, even apart from a nutritionally excellent meal?

Sandy introduces our speaker, Lanette D. Young, a registered dietitian with The Heart Institute of St. Petersburg, and we clap politely. Lanette picks up her control for the computer which will project her slides and launches right in.

"One out of two American men will die of heart disease and one out of two women as well—just later, after menopause. And yet, this is a *preventible* disease and, if you have it, it's *manageable.*" She smiles.

"What are the symptoms of high cholesterol?" she asks.

"There aren't any!" several oldsters reply.

"Ah, you've heard that one before," Lanette continues brightly. "You're right. There are no symptoms . . . you can't guess your own numbers . . . you can't feel anything. Only a screening—an actual blood test—will tell you what you're pumping around your body."

She goes on to explain the major plasma lipids—forms of fat that float in our blood. There are three major forms of plasma lipids, which are bound to proteins for transport, hence the name lipoprotein: the triglycerides, high-density cholesterol (HDL), and low-density cholesterol (LDL). The triglycerides are many and active, depending largely on what we've eaten lately. Blood testing, therefore, is most accurate when you've been fasting. If you eat a stick of butter—ninety-six grams of fat, some nine hundred calories—your intestines will absorb it into your blood stream, and your blood plasma (that is, the liquid without the red or white cells) will turn butter colored with all the fat. If you're a sled-dog in Alaska running the Iditarod race, you'd happily gobble down frozen sticks of butter, and your heroic physical expenditure would burn these right up. (Also, dogs don't get obstructive heart disease.) In general, what you eat goes directly or indirectly (after digestion) into your blood and through your heart and arteries; that's the only way it can get to all the cells to nourish them. Heart and vasculature are the highway for everything we eat. Thus there's a nutritional truth in the phrase "taking something to heart." Your body is the "downstream" to whatever you eat. I think of the weight-loss slogan "A moment on the lips, a lifetime on the hips." What might a parallel cardiac version be? Perhaps "Everything you swallow affects your arteries, which you want to keep hollow."

I remember watching an autopsy of an eighty-year-old woman. The doctor, a pathology resident, had removed the descending aorta. When she sliced down it and opened it up, it was white and clean inside, no atheromas. Her attending physician—an outgoing Texan—was observing from the other side of the stainless steel table. "OOO-EEE!" he exclaimed. "I'd trade for that in an eyeblink!"

Lanette tells us that fats give *satiety,* a sense of satisfaction. There are two aspects to this. Food engineers speak of "mouthfeel" to describe the smooth, creamy texture of ice cream and the warm, juicy sensation of steak, as well as many other upscale foods, pastries, sauced dishes, and desserts. "A nice, juicy steak," we say, ignoring that the juice, when refrigerated, turns to white globs of fat. Probably our natural history taught us to enjoy the mouthfeel of fat so that we'd seek it out in nature, which is poor in fat. Today, however, fat is a tidal wave in the diets of developed—that is, rich—countries. (Indeed, we speak of fat-laden food as being "rich.") The second sense of satiety is a filling sensation in our guts. My mother used to say, "Steak and potatoes [with gravy, cheese, sour cream, and/or butter] sticks to your ribs," meaning that fatty foods stay longer in the gut and hunger is slower to return. (Some diplomats used to eat butter before going to cocktail parties in order to slow absorption of alcohol.) Low-fat Chinese meals have been criticized in the United States for not staving off hunger adequately: "an hour later you're hungry!" But Chinese cuisine is one of the healthiest.

I think of strawberry season in Florida, which is in March. It's the only time my wife and I buy those nifty cans of whipped cream for strawberry shortcake. The sweet white stuff comes out in lovely fluted patterns. There's a satisfying noise. Pent-up demand seizes me and I squirt the cream onto my hand and lick it off. Delicious! Cool, sweet, tinged with vanilla—but the label on the can tells me 75 percent of its calories come from fat which will soon swirl in my veins, my arteries, my heart. We need some fat in our diets, of course, and some fat in our bodies. Fat is an ideal way to store calories, important for humans when food is (or was—as we saw earlier) scarce. Pregnant women need to store enough fat to fuel them while they are pregnant and while they care for their babies. (Men on the lookout for women always, by instinct, look for adequate fat stores.) Subdermal fat helps keep us warm. Fat cushions our internal organs: even a healthy heart has fat on the pericardium. But some 50 to 60 percent of Americans are over ideal weights; stadium seats have been made wider, and clothing sizes inch upward. The most frequently named reasons for our collective bulk are fatty diets, high total caloric intake, and sedentary lifestyles—sitting at desks, watching TV, riding in cars. But I know from my own instances of overeating that there are other psychological factors, including hunger for immediate reward (the refrigerator light comes on to greet me!), boredom, or a ritual pleasure of comfort foods—all of which suggest emptiness that I attempt to fill up with food.

Lanette shows a slide contrasting a fast-food meal and a brown-bag lunch. The fast-food meal is a hamburger, french fries, a soft drink, and a milkshake. Who'd want a soft drink *and* a shake, I wonder, but the numbers make her point clear: the fast-food lunch totals 2,200 calories, a typical number for a man for an entire day, well over the 1,800 a woman typically needs. The fat picture is even grimmer: ninety-six grams, which equals one stick of butter, well over the fifty-five to sixty grams a person needs, a day and a half's worth, in fact. And of this, much is saturated fat—the worst kind. On the other side of the slide is a turkey sandwich, a carrot, a carton of low-fat milk, and an apple. It totals 350 calories with only 6 grams of fat!

The next slide shows a cartoon of a man holding the food pyramid upside down, and a doctor trying to turn it right side up. The man wants to eat the typical American diet, high in fats, salt, refined foods. The food pyramid was created in 1992 by the U.S. Food and Drug Administration and the Department of Health and Human Services to increase the traditional food groups from four to six and to illustrate graphically the proportions we should be eating. More grains, fruits, and vegetables. Less dairy, meat, and, especially, fats, oils, and sweets, pictured in the uppermost, tiny triangle. This is a diet that eats "lower on the food chain," as many have said and, in terms of the natural history of the human race, closer to the way our forebears ate for millennia. As one speaker put it, "If you go into nature, what will you eat, assuming you have the knowledge and ability to gather and catch your food? Danish pastries? Milkshakes? Anything refined?" In more recent times "non-developed" cultures still consume grains and vegetables for the most part, and high cholesterol—and heart disease—are rare.

Thirteen years later, the USDA brought out a new pyramid, modishly entitled MyPyramid. This design shows a set of steps up the left side, where a stylized human figure jogs upward two steps at a time. Instead of the previous building blocks within the pyramid, there are now six paths of different colors starting from the bottom and tapering to the point on top. Furthermore, the pyramid is dynamic: different sizes for different folks; you can access them all at www.mypyramid.gov. Thus the search continues for the best image to mo-tivate Americans, complete now with an electronic dimension on the Internet, interactive for today's audience. Still, experts have complained, "Where's the food?" (see *Food & Fitness Advisor* Aug. 7, July 2005: 9), because the new pyramid paths are not labeled, nor is there advice about what foods not to eat. A deeper question might be: why should Americans want to jog up any pyramid?

Two of the three numbers in the cholesterol profile are the high-density and the low-density lipoproteins. Since only animals produce cholesterol, we get it in our diet only by eating such foods as meats or egg yolks. Products like peanut butter cannot, by the nature of peanuts, have any cholesterol. (Still, marketers will blazon "No Cholesterol" on vegetable products, banking on the lack of knowledge of consumers; they might as well label watermelons as having "No Bones!") Peanut butter can, however, be laden with corn syrup and saturated fats—another sad story.

The LDLs, or low-density lipoproteins, are the bad guys. Lanette says, "Just remember the first 'L' is for 'lousy.'" LDLs, especially if too high, can build up on artery walls and eventually cause heart attacks. I know that I'm borderline high for my cholesterol total (230 mg/ml) and have been so for years. Despite sporadic efforts to control this number, it's stayed pretty constant. I know that my doctor has muttered that my LDLs are higher than he'd like to see, but I've never paid any lasting attention to the number. He says exercise is the best way to lower them, as well as, of course, eating right. The "good" ones, the other ones, are the HDLs, highly-density lipoproteins. Lanette tells us that the "H" can be remembered as standing for "healthy" because they clear away some of the LDLs sticking on cell walls which can lead to restriction of blood flow.

It's good to have a reading of 40 or even 50 for HDLs, but 60 or 70 is better. Indeed, the higher the better; people who live to be a hundred or more have very high HDL levels (80 to 100), which appear to be caused by a recently discovered gene, aptly called the "Methuselah gene." Typically, Lanette says, smoking knocks off 10 points of a person's HDL values. What are mine? I have no idea. I vow to write down the whole lipid profile number at my next health check; since I always carry a calendar, I can put the numbers on a page in the back as reminders, as comparisons for future readings. Total cholesterol is the sum of HDLs, LDLs, and VLDLs (very-low-density lipoproteins); a reading below 200 is desirable.

The danger levels for LDL correlates with other risk factors (being a male over forty-five, a female over fifty-five, a female under fifty-five who has had a hysterectomy but no hormone replacement, family history of heart disease, smoking, high blood pressure, diabetes). With one risk factor, you want to be under 160 for LDL. With two risk factors, you want to be below 130. With actual heart disease, you want to be at or below 100. Heart patients become very concerned with these numbers; in a sense, their lives depend on them. (Since this talk, some of these numbers have been revised downward; we should get the latest word from our physicians as medical information continues to evolve.)

The first line of therapy for persons whose levels are too high are behavioral: stop smoking, control drinking and diet, and exercise. If these efforts do not lower the numbers enough (or if patients don't actually do them), drugs are the next approach. Some of these pills cost ninety dollars a bottle . . . and can have side effects. I resolve to watch what I eat and to be more faithful in exercising.

What can a "heart-healthy" diet do for a person? It can lower a person's weight. It can lower blood pressure, which causes wear and tear on the heart and vasculature. It can help prevent diabetes or help control it in diabetic patients. It can help prevent cancer. It can make stretching and exercising easier. It can improve one's self-image. It can promote emotional health. Judging from my meal tonight, it can give feelings of joy and personal control about "eating right."

And eating all the bad stuff? What is the emptiness we try to fill with alcohol, fats, salt, too many calories? Why do we need "comfort foods," many of which are not good for us; why do we gobble fat-laden, salt-laden fast food?

As I leave the church parking lot, I realize that there is a concrete sense in which you can *eat your heart out,* but I also know there are some factors we cannot control. I remember a woman who "did everything right," but still had high cholesterol, owing to her genes. She was a rare case, of course, but she also presented a good model for all of us: that we should do the best we can with whatever genes we have inherited.

Do You Like Mangoes?

I pay a second call on the Reddicks to show them how I wrote up our interview and to get their approval and any corrections. We sit as before in the television room, Johnnie in his recliner, with his feet up.

"How do you feel?" I ask.

"I feel fine, although I'm weak," he says.

We talk about his health and what I wrote. We also talk about the recent disappearance of John F. Kennedy Jr.'s airplane and the three passengers aboard. Indeed the whole nation is focused on this story, because—at least in part—it represents some version of gratuitous death. If famous people can be so plucked from life, what hope is there for the rest of us?

"JFK was one of my favorite presidents," Johnnie says. "I remember he reviewed some troops and asked why there were no black persons in the ranks. The next year we were there." I think of Michael's interest in Arnold Schwarzenegger as a protector, a symbolic intercessor.

"Do you like mangoes?" Zelma asks.

"Yes," I say. My wife and I have been buying them steadily this summer. The succulent, richly flavored flesh is a treat well worth the difficulty of cutting the fruit away from its large flat seed. According to the newspaper, mangoes are quite popular this year, and people in Florida are buying trees of different varieties to plant at home, even on condo porches.

Zelma goes to the garage and returns with a plastic shopping bag loaded with maybe a dozen mangoes. It's quite heavy . . . and smells wonderful.

Johnnie chips in, "We have so many, she could sell them. But we give them away to neighbors, at church, and so on."

"Are these ready to eat?"

"Oh yes. They're ready when they fall off the tree. Besides, I don't like them mushy. Falling down is a sign they're ready," she says.

As I drive home, the odor of ripe mangoes fills the car. *Falling down is a sign they're ready* rings in my head. At his age Johnnie can't have much more time ahead of him. And yet very sick people—who fall down one way or another—often stand up to live. I think of my wife's burst appendix and her recovery. The hospice guideline for offering care is that death is likely within six months; no doctor can calculate this exactly, of course (unlike the closer calculation possible for pregnancy). Furthermore, readiness for death is not a fashionable notion in this culture currently. We'd rather live what Tolstoy's character Ivan Ilyich called "the Lie," that we're all going to live a long time and in terrific health. Anyone who is sick or near death is a challenge, a threat to our story of optimal life. If we see persons with debility in public places, we've been taught to look away, presumably out of sympathy with them, but perhaps also because they bring us news we don't want to accept, including the possibility that someday any of us might be like them.

I have learned today that my secretary at work has been referred to hospice because her cancer will probably give her only three to six months of life. I know she wanted to work another ten months to get her retirement benefits. Further, a son of a fellow professor—his office is across the hall from mine—has drowned in the college swimming pool. He was fifteen. I think of the tragedy for this family . . . and for the lifeguard. (Many years ago I was a guard in that pool myself; I would have been shattered if one of the swimmers I was guarding had died during my watch.) A week ago, I sang at a memorial service for Wilhelmina Rowland Smith, a redoubtable woman who died at ninety-one. And the John F. Kennedy Jr. disaster . . .

When the mangoes are ripe, they fall from the tree. When an older person dies, especially if they are in pain or debility, we can accept it more readily than when it's a younger person. Death . . . the great absurdity, especially for most Americans. How far off is Johnnie's death? No one knows, of course, but when it comes it seems certain that he and Zelma will be more ready than many of us.

Feeding Our Hearts (Fourth Essay)

I keep thinking about Dylan in the emergency room. Despite his cough and obvious physical discomfort, he seemed calm, at ease. His faith was deep; he generously shared it with me. I felt a contrast with how I was raised; coming from a non-evangelical background, I was taught to live a faith but not to proselytize. In America, for several reasons, many of us keep our faiths hidden, especially in these "politically correct" times, but also in many decades before. Church and state were held to be separate, and daily secular life and any religious impulses were often held separate; further, respect for other people's views often meant that we did not mention our own. Like Michael's fellow students at Stanford, we are so careful not to mention faith that it is often taboo, an aspect of life that would be embarrassing to mention. Indeed, we have a schizophrenia of sorts regarding religion: polls of Americans show that many believe in God and an afterlife and that many have religious interests and spiritual needs; at the same time, numbers of churchgoers are falling in many denominations, and public discourse on religious matters appears in narrow channels, such as academic writing. And, of course, many have no overtly religious faith, although they usually believe in some set of overarching values, however implicit. Most Americans have been largely affirming of some higher truths, even with the doubts and fears following September 11, 2001, but we are reluctant to state our deepest beliefs, religious or not, consciously held or not. But Dylan, sick in his ER bed, says "It is easy" to see things in terms of *yes* with a trust in God. We stamp our coins "In God we trust," but our intellectual lives are usually rational and our economic lives Darwinian and competitive.

Our culture (and education, and mass media) is saturated with rationalism, science, objective proofs, logic, cause-and-effect reasoning, Newtonian thinking, and the like. Early in the twentieth century, the Cambridge anthropologists, such as G. F. Frazier, felt that religion was a primitive aspect of society, and that the moderns had clearly moved on to science. But such science—as useful as it was in many ways—gave a flattened view of the world and of human nature, throwing out emotions, intuition, paradox, and mystery. While the twentieth-century physics of Einstein, Heisenberg, Feynman, Hawking, and others re-introduced uncertainty, relativism, and the subjectivism of the viewer, much of the culture at large held with the earlier, linear rationalism. Pragmatism, practicality, and Yankee common sense are as American as apple pie. Missouri calls itself the "Show Me" state, where you don't take anything on faith.

In contrast, the romantics, whether European or American, held that the inner, emotional life was rich, true, and in tune with nature. In *The Prelude*, the young Wordsworth borrows a rowboat for an unauthorized ride and feels in his inner being that he is wrong and that the surrounding mountains are coming after him. Feelings, personal meanings, intuitions—these are ignored by education so that we can "fit in" with corporate, rational, industrial America. The Myers-Briggs test uses the polarity of "sensing" versus "intuition," finding that three-fourths of Americans would rather measure, count, and touch to gain knowledge than by a sudden flash of recognition and insight. Both means are necessary, of course, for a person, a business, a nation, but the latter is currently out of favor in a rational culture. And so are the "heart's reasons" of Pascal, and the "habits of the heart" of Bellah.

As a result, we often feel that we should hide the traditional heart values, our emotions, our feelings, our intuitions—especially if we are Real Men, as Steve Oreskovich found. And we should make fun of flakes, hippies, artists, enviros, granolas, tree huggers, and the like, calling them narcissists, solipsists, the self-absorbed and self-indulgent.

If you rule such capacities out of bounds, what do you get? Hunger, American style. A culture that suppresses emotions, religion, and personal intuitions becomes not only hungry but also bored. Its members try different strategies to survive. Some focus on wealth and material goods, such as cars, houses, and clothes. Some seek social status in the right clubs, the top schools for their children, expensive travel. Some become obsessive workers. (Robert Kugelman's argument is that our grief over the loss of nature, loss of neighborhoods, loss of leisure time has been translated—engineered, he says—into obsessive work habits.) Some take drugs. Some overeat, drink, smoke, or shop. Are these not the marks of a decadent culture, where jaded people seek continuous and novel stimulation to make themselves happy? Computer games. Special effects in movies. Two hundred channels on cable TV. The Internet. Where can we find the satiety Lanette spoke of in our mouths, in our guts, in our lives?

Nourishment comes in many forms, of course. At the literal level, certain foodstuffs keep us alive; Lanette spoke of good diets to nourish the body and protect the heart. Good cooks know how to make dishes attractive; good hosts know how to welcome guests, make them feel comfortable. I was pleased that Nurse Giles brought me a milkshake. The nourishment of a symbol (the street person's Sacred Heart of Jesus), of human touch, of prayer (as George found), or a loving gesture of a bag of mangoes takes away some of our hungers and our fears by giving us an image to which we can relate sensuously; such images can provide us with meaning, connection with other persons, and a wider context than our current troubles. For religious persons such as George and the street person, symbolic nourishment can take many forms. Johnnie likes it when Reverend Terry brings him communion; I appreciated the company and prayers of my minister in the emergency room. The word "nourishment" has several cousins, all with the same Latin root, in "nursing," "nursery," "nursing home," which have specialized into the various realms of sick people, infants, and oldsters. Certainly such people need nourishment, but so does everyone else. Nurses help the sick and the very young and the very old, but ideally it should be all of us nursing/nourishing everyone else through language, gifts, kind acts, symbolic acts. "Commit random acts of kindness" reads a recent bumper sticker, a plea for a more loving society.

One college where I taught rearranged classes so that there was no longer a common lunch hour when various communities—professors, staff, administrators, students—could eat together. The loss of social ecology (Bellah's phrase) was never measured—nor could be, I expect, but persons who worked under both systems could tell the difference in the loss of colleagueship, exchange of personal news, and morale. Conflict resolution specialists know that one effective tool is this: serve food to the parties assembled. (Once I went to a lunch meeting with some difficult issues to resolve. Our leader served food, but one of the participants refused to eat, signaling his intransigence.) Cultures of many times and places serve food and drink to show hospitality: mint tea in Morocco, the tea ceremony in Japan. God gave the wandering Hebrews manna in the desert (Exodus 16). When Jesus offers the Samaritan woman at the well the water of eternal life, she asks him to give it to her (John 4:13–15). The Christian communion connects worshipers with God, with each other, and with two thousand years of tradition.

I'm thinking about the angels in the living room of the Reddicks. Traditionally, angels shuttle back and forth between heaven and earth, connecting our physical and spiritual lives; indeed the Greek root *angelos* means *messenger*. In mythic terms, they are a personified axis mundi, an avenue of connection between heaven and earth, much like Jacob's ladder or the vertical dimension of the Christian cross. A related concept is the *psychopomp,* the guide of souls (psyche) in a procession (pomp) at death, leading us upward from earth to heaven. According to Herder's *Guide to Symbols,* numerous cultures have a version of psychopomps (be they chickens, jaguars, apes, reindeer, or dolphins), but especially for Christians: angels. At the end of *Hamlet,* Horatio says, "Goodnight sweet prince, / And flights of angels sing thee to thy rest!" In Goethe's *Faust,* cherubs throw roses at the Devil to confuse him, then whisk Faust's soul away to heaven. In spirituals, images of angels (as in the song "Swing Low, Sweet Chariot") or Jesus himself as guides to heaven are commonplace. Despite the sudden popularity of angels in the last few years, even religious people in this society don't typically have an image of angels as guardian spirits that carry us to heaven. We are more likely to hear of relatives in white waving to us at the other end of the tunnel (my father had such a vision in a near-death episode), but personal guides—as Virgil was for Dante—seem to have faded away. This loss of connection between this world and the next is another loss (like the loss of nature) that contributes to a pervasive sense of anomie, rootlessness, meaninglessness. With no prospects of welcome to the next world, we must go for all the gusto in this one.

Losing a sense of hosts from the next world may also contribute to our loss of being hosts in this one. In cities people don't drop by to sit on the porch and visit, as was common when I was growing up in 1940s and 1950s Arkansas. The arts of gossip, loaning tools and recipes, exchanging clothes, barn raisings, or other community projects are in decline, again isolating us further. The exceptions to my claim—shared gardens, co-ops, street cleanups, Habitat for Humanity construction—can be very satisfying and heartening to a community.

Another traditional link to the heavens has been smoke. The psalmist declared, "Let my prayer be counted as incense before you, and the lifting up of my hands as an evening sacrifice," (Psalms 141:2); incense and other sacrifices were burned on an altar, a platform symbolically half way between earth and heaven, a meeting place of the two realms, and the smoke rising a stairway to heaven in the tradition of the axis mundi (as in Jacob's ladder). A more modern version is George Croly's nineteenth-century hymn, "Spirit of God, Descend Upon My Heart," which concludes with this stanza:

> Teach me to love Thee as Thine angels love,
> One holy passion filling all my frame;
> The baptism of the heaven-descended Dove.
> My heart an altar, and Thy love the flame.

In Croly's vision, the divine enters our hearts as vital energy symbolized by the dove which connects heaven and earth, yet another version of the axis mundi. Croly's poem emphasizes the mystical link between "my heart" and the Godhead, but others have suggested that such a link finds expression in love shown to others humans ("We love because he first loved us," 1 John 4:19), or the horizontal dimension of the Christian cross, a radiating love, much like the street person's image of the Sacred Heart of Jesus. I think of a couple of non-Christians, Baucis and Philemon, lovingly described by Ovid in his *Metamorphoses* (Bk. VIII). An aging couple, they are loving to each other and to traveling guests. One day Zeus and Hermes in disguise stop by, having been denied hospitality by others time after time. Baucis and Philemon take them in and, despite their modest means, offer them a meal. Their generosity is echoed by a supernatural event: the bowl of wine continuously refills itself. The gods ask the aged couple what reward they should like and, in one translation, they reply, our "hearts' desire" is to take care of a temple and not outlive each other. (Although *cor* does not appear in the Latin, this translation is true to the characters and the events.) The poem celebrates generosity of hosts and faithfulness of couples, two clear values of the heart, two values I found when I visited Johnnie and Zelma Reddick.

I have heard sermons with the following allegory of nourishment when persons eat together; it may be a very old story—I've been told there is a version in a Hasidic tale: a recently dead person goes to Limbo for judgment and a speedy trip to Heaven or Hell. There he's given a long spoon, longer than his arm. His hand is attached to the end. "Hey," he protests, "I can't get this to my mouth!" At that moment a window opens up to show Hell, where angry sinners are surrounded by tables of wonderful food. Because of the length of their spoons, however, they can eat none of it. "Does this mean I'm going to Hell?" he asks, holding up his spoon. Another window opens up, this one on Heaven. Here are the same tables, but many happy people. They have the same spoons. They are feeding each other.

In the Bible, the phrase a "host of angels" means that the angels were servants of God, attending him (or her). The notion of service survives in a phrase "ancillary personnel," used for nurses and medical techs. It's a somewhat condescending phrase that is slowly disappearing in favor of the phrase "allied health professionals." The root is the Latin word "ancilla," or "maid." If the phrase has any helpful meaning, it would be that *all* health-care personnel, doctors included, should be ancillary to the lives of their patients.

The street person carried the emblem of the Sacred Heart of Jesus foremost in his wallet, the first thing he saw whenever he opened it, feeding his heart. He had no physical house but a spiritual home. What is the quality of our mental space? Is it fearful or thankful? Hungry or nourished? The imagination is powerful, as any of us know from waking in the middle of the night and reviewing our anxieties, our hurts, our fears. George's doctors did wonderful surgery on him; they saved his life. But his cultural heart (we might say) still needed a healing that a laying on of hands could provide. As the Hebrews put it long ago, "A cheerful heart is good medicine, but a downcast spirit dries up the bones" (Proverbs 17:22). A crucial point in the Catholic mass is the exclamation, "Sursum corda," or "Lift up your hearts." Conversely, as Johnnie Reddick put it, "It's the devil that's afraid."

Western medicine is now in conversation with alternative medicine; indeed we hear the phrases "complementary medicine," even "integrative medicine" and "ecological medicine" to describe new overlaps and symbioses. Medical schools now have courses in alternative medicine, and national research is giving alternative therapies careful study to see whether or to what extent they work; if efficacy is proved in western terms, traditional doctors will be more likely in the future to work with yoga, acupuncture, massage, music, herbal medicine, and spirituality. As our culture is less bound by the positivism of the nineteenth century, we are now more open to considering wider realms of healing. The menu of foods to nourish the heart becomes more generous, more varied, and, I hope, more satisfying.

There are radical dimensions that are alarming, however. If we take ecological medicine seriously, we would have to take the health of our environment seriously, understanding that humans are part of nature. We'd have to control pollution of all kinds, petrochemicals, nuclear waste, and some (some say all) aspects of genetic engineering. We'd have to control medical waste which, when incinerated, provides one of the largest sources of dioxin. (See, on the Web, Bioneers, Science and Environmental Health Network, and the Center for Health, Environment and Justice.) Are these New Age concerns, or is living in tune with nature part of an Old Age we should return to? Can we head "forward" to some of the things we recently forgot but nonetheless keep the advantages of modern knowledge and technology?

When I was an undergraduate I became captivated by rationalism. My upbringing had included Protestant worship and Sunday school, both of which—when I reached college—suddenly seemed jejune. Surely the mind could perceive all, analyze all, and sufficiently prescribe and control so that life would be clear and orderly. I decided I had outgrown matters of faith, the transcendent, and the phony and judgmental trappings of the church; I became a nonbeliever. In the next half dozen years, I married, my father died of brain cancer, and the United States became involved in Vietnam, where men known to me died, where I too might have been sent, had I not been a student. Suddenly the world was not as susceptible to rational perception or analysis. I still loved the mind, but I came to honor once again a spiritual life and found joy and comfort in private prayer and in communal worship.

As much as I have studied the physical, biological heart, it does not eclipse for me the cultural heart, the heart of love, the erotic, and the spiritual. Ancient religions have seen the heart as a meeting place of the human and the divine, and for some people this may still be a powerful notion. If God (or the gods), working through nature, gave us the magnificent gifts of our hearts, we can celebrate them and be joyful. Instead of wondering when my heart is going to betray me, I may be thankful for it and consider that its four chambers provide space, not just for blood, but for all the higher faculties of spirits, angels, and divine beings I may host there. If I consider it a banquet hall, then it is I who serve my guests. And perhaps they will bring something too. But I need not demand nourishment for my heart; by nourishing others, I too will be fed.

While the heart, for some persons, is a place of holiness, a place to meet the divine, I do not consider religion the only way we can be "hearted." One etymology for "religion" suggests that it ties things together, like a ligature. Surely other synthetic and holistic worldviews can nourish us, whether they are forms of animism, vitalism, humanism, nature worship, or something else. I'm thinking of heart values in the widest sense: sympathy, love, respect, affirmation, sharing, cooperation, admiration, appreciation, kindness, joy, enlightenment, and mystery. While we still have a hundred heart phrases, our society is slow to affirm the heart values implied, to celebrate them, to teach them to our young, and to affirm people and institutions who put them into practice. I'd like to see the motto "Practice random acts of kindness" in more places than on an occasional bumper sticker. Affirming and practicing such heart values, it seems to me, would lower stress and raise, both corporately and individually, our sense of being nourished. Better nourished, we would need fewer toys and baubles, and we might be able to eat less and enjoy nature more.

One spring my wife Nancy and I met another couple, Marian and Tommy Price, on the Ridge, a central spine of the Florida peninsula that includes its highest elevation, all 392 feet above sea level. This Lake Wales Ridge is covered with wonderful white sand, a product of a distant time when "Florida" was only some twenty-five to fifty miles wide, a narrow strip surrounded by seas that crashed on the shore and ground up the limestone. (At other times, this peninsula was very wide, when glaciers locked up much of earth's water; like the heart, this land has contracted and expanded.) Today, the Ridge is largely developed for towns, highways, some cattle ranches, and acre upon acre of orange groves. Little first-growth forest is still available, but the state park Highlands Hammock is one such area.

There are a series of paths through immense live oaks through which slender palms snake their trunks up and up so that their fronds can feel the sun. There are some pioneer buildings and some pines that were slashed long ago to harvest pitch. One walkway goes through a cypress marsh, where we saw an alligator floating. On another boardwalk we heard eager, high-pitched cries. We moved up and down the boardwalk, trying in vain to find the nest in the woods perhaps fifty to sixty feet away. Then we heard a similar cry, but louder, longer, and at a lower pitch, as an adult red-tailed hawk landed in a tree just thirty feet ahead of us. This mother (we assumed) had something in her sharp, curved beak. Her large eye blinked. She and her nestlings called back and forth for a few minutes before she unfurled her wings and flew into the woods to the nest.

In another area of the oldest and largest live oaks we heard a nearby *gobble gobble* that we assumed was a wild turkey. We advanced slowly and quietly down our trail, peering into the palmettos but finding nothing. A flash of red off to the side caught my eye, however, and my binoculars found an adult pileated woodpecker landing in the fork of a dead pine tree. Such snags are common nesting sites for woodpeckers, providing insects for food and shelter for young in hollowed-out cavities; pileateds are now our largest woodpecker, up to twenty inches in length. One bird book calls them "spectacular." As I lowered the glasses to give them to Nancy, other red shapes appeared to be moving.

"Pileated . . . a big one. And a mate?" I whispered.

"No . . . babies!" Nancy exclaimed.

Sure enough, four red-crested nestlings jumped around in their wooden cavern, jockeying for food from good old Mom. She served them in turn, dipping her beak into theirs, lowering her head with its dramatic red crest like a flame. As we passed the binoculars back and forth, mother pileated fed both her young and four middle-aged voyeurs. I thought of William Blake's line, "For every thing that lives is Holy," with the emphasis on the word *lives*.

Turning to our alcove model, we can fill in the last quadrant. Johnnie and Zelma represent persons for whom the heart is home of the spirit. While they turn to standard medical care for Johnnie's heart problems (including Zelma's nursing of him at home), they also supplement with prayer, religious belief and practice, images (such as angels), and shark cartilage. Even in my brief time with them, I can see that a loving relationship, the symbolism of food (water and mangoes offered to me), and the protective spirits of angels are important as well. The angels were placed on a special table in the living room, a symbolic altar, we might say. For this couple I'll suggest that the functional metaphor for the heart is, indeed, an altar, a meeting place for humans and the divine.

Alcove Model: Four Perspectives on the Heart

a. Person
b. A biological definition of heart
c. Diagnosed illness(es)

d. Branch of treating medicine
e. Medical intervention(s)
f. Patient concept(s) of heart
g. Patient support strategies

h. Humanistic perspective
i. Outcome aim
j. Exemplary metaphor

a. **Michael**
b. Hemodynamic organ
c. Incompetent valve
d. Cardiac surgery
e. Ross procedure
f. Basis for life, athletics
g. Rehab, family, friends, words
h. Words, naming of parts
i. Healthy valves
j. Gift

a. **Steve**
b. Vulnerable to stress
c. Coronary artery disease
d Interventional radiology
e. Angioplasty/stress reduction
f . Stressed; locus of feeling
g. Counseling, behavioral changes
h. Implicit stories
i. Clean coronary arteries
j. Partner

**OUR
HUMAN
HEART**

a. **Kay**
b. Biochemical wonder
c. Viral cardiomyopathy
d. Cardiology, internal medicine
e. Pharmaceuticals

f. A wild animal to ride, to manage
g. Friends, yoga, rodeos, counseling
h. Stories
i. Adequate ejection fraction
j. Miracle

a. **Johnnie**
b. Vulnerable to high blood pressure
c. Various (stroke, failure, arrhythmia)
d. Various, Cardiology
e. Various, pharmaceuticals,
   cardioversion
f. Home of spirit
g. Prayer, alternative medicine
h. Images (angels), symbolic food
i. Adequate circulation
j. Altar

Alcove Model showing four perspectives of the heart. The Reddicks give us another way of perceiving the heart. Although this drawing has a seductive parallel to the four chambers of the mammalian heart, other perspectives (genetic, bioenergetic, environmental) might be proposed, and still others will surely emerge in the future, as models of medicine and health care evolve.

Our Human Hearts

OUR VIEWS of the heart are an evolving cultural artifact, created over a very long time, perhaps as long as humans could communicate meanings of any sort. Why is this so? The first reason, of course, is that the heart has been seen as central to life for millennia, a sine qua non for our very lives. The ancients knew nothing of gaseous exchanges or neurohumoral factors, but they surely knew that a beating heart meant life and a still heart meant death—basic meanings that we still appreciate. The second reason is that humans are, par excellence, the interpretive animal; to be human is to be hermeneutic, to wrest meanings from (or to cast meanings upon) objects, concepts, fellow creatures, and portions of our own bodies. The ancient world (at least in the West) didn't perceive the brain as very interesting; the genitals seem largely cloaked by taboo. In between the two, the heart was clearly central in the body and inter- preted as central to human existence, physically, emotionally, and spiritually, as we have seen. The heart is a basic organ that helps, by its steady beating, to define our humanity from within. The heart has fascinated us for millennia, a modest, strange-looking lump of flesh upon which we have projected a wide variety of meanings that define us, once again, as humans, those creatures who persistently—obsessively, we might even say—seek meanings. Such meanings may be scientific, religious, alchemical, literary, athletic, cultural, or of many other sorts. Thus the heart is a sort of a mirror or Rorschach blot, reflecting some of our basic concerns or interpretive strategies. We project upon it some of the dominant notions of any given generation, whether the image of a mechanical pump, the canary in the mine shaft, or an organ replaceable by another heart or even a high-tech device; some of these notions change with larger trends of intellectual history or fashions of the day; some of these are colored by traditions of faith, as in the Sacred Heart of Jesus.

In my case, I started this study with a fear, the neurotic definition of my mortal heart as a betrayer within, a storage place for my anxieties. An heir of my grandmother's heart disease, my heart was surely capable of ambush and assassination. This strange definition haunted me as a game to spice up my life, in part a facile and paranoid use of a target of opportunity, in part an internalization of media reports about stress and heart illness. And yet these values were not readily apparent to me: I played the game at a subconscious level, a series of implicit metaphors that had to be raised into explicit consciousness, brought to clear definition so that I could exorcize them and replace them with other metaphors that were more helpful, calming, affirming, even healing. Am I healed completely? Did I lift up the Antaeus of my anxieties and, Hercules-like, strangle him? Probably not. Life still has stresses; I'm still mildly hypochondriac. I will likely find other target organs or body systems to interpret negatively. I may return to my heart as an easy cubby to stuff my fears in, especially if I have any kind of chest pain. But I can be more aware of these cheap tricks and of how to deal with my fears. I also have faith in western medicine to help me with a wide range of accidents and illness, including cardiac disease. I will not die alone in a car on a street, unwilling to seek help—as my Uncle Hector almost did years ago in downtown Chicago, while hundreds of people swirled past him and medical help was but a 911 call away. Luckily for him, a passerby saw him white and sweating, slumped over the steering wheel, and she (or he—we never knew which) called for help and—in all probability—saved his life.

How many hearts do we have? The question seems silly given that each of us has one single, physical heart and that it is roughly the same as the heart in every other person. We speak of "the heart" as an existential absolute, but, as we have seen, it mirrors two aspects of our consciousness, the cultural and the biomedical. The cultural heart is various and multiple, given different cultures, different centuries, different expressive media, and so on. As for the physical, biological heart, doctors transplant them every day, don't they? Yet there's a narrow range of acceptable organs—those matching by size, blood type, and HLA (human leukocyte antigens) factors—not to mention narrow range of availability upon someone else's death, since we can't (or can't yet) store hearts like automotive parts.

As biological entities, hearts are only roughly the same from person to person, only roughly the same for each of us throughout our lives. (In my fifties I saw an X-ray of my chest and heard my doctor say, "Look at that broadening aorta; it's OK, but it does show your age.") Further, anyone who has been successfully treated for heart disease knows at least three hearts—the previously healthy one, the initially sick one, and the one that has evolved since then, for better or worse. People training aerobically will often see their resting pulse rate slowly drop, as their hearts become more efficient. (When I was a long-distance runner, my waking pulse was as low as 43 bpm; twenty years later—with moderate walking for exercise it's more like 63). We can even consider a given heart in a given week, say, to exist in a wide range of states, from the slow beats of profound rest to the rapid pulse accompanying maximal effort;

yes, it's the same organ, but it has different ways of being as our activities and mental states change. And, over a lifetime, a given heart exists in many ways, from its first pulsatile waves about day twenty-two in the tiny embryo to its last beats at death. One simple definition of the heart is *the blood-pumping organ that supports our lives through its durability and synthetic multiplicity.* The first part of the definition (up through "supports our lives") emphasizes the basic, simple fact that we owe our lives to our heart's basic functions; this fact is of prime importance to heart patients, while healthy persons usually take it for granted. The second part of the definition moves us toward two possible observations.

The first—durability—is well known, a virtue we see celebrated in various clichés: "Slow and steady wins the race," "Hang in there!" and even "He who laughs last laughs best." Sometimes this concept is broken down into doable units: "A journey of a thousand miles begins with a single step." "I'll worry only about today; yesterday is gone, tomorrow will take care of itself," and the like. Or Woody Allen's, "Half of success is just showing up." We can see reflected in our hearts the quality of persistence. The word "faithful" may be too per-sonified, too sentimental a quality to project upon hearts (as in a pet dog), but our hearts do keep working, and keep on working in a way that we can count on, usually for decades, even when we often don't take care of them well. We could say they mark (if not measure—as in the song "Grandfather's Clock") our journeys one beat at a time. When they finally give out, the reasons are sometimes attributable to our care of them and sometimes not. At least for me, considering the heart's wondrous durability inspires me to want to support it through good health habits—as regularly as I care for my teeth. Not only is it my partner, as we saw in Steve's section, but I can be its partner.

The second observation—synthetic multiplicity—is more complex and speculative. We've seen that the heart works with every bodily system: vascular (blood circulation), bones (blood cells' origin), muscles (nourishment and gaseous exchanges via the blood), neurological and hormonal (controlling the heart's speed and volume), gastrointestinal (blood transportation of food products), genitourinary (filters blood), and our organs of special sense (such as our eyes) and even our skin, all of which need blood supply to survive and function. The tentative conclusions I draw are twofold. First, taking the heart as an inspiring image of synthesis, we can enrich our lives through varied in-terests and activities. As one cliché has it, "No one retiring says, 'Boy, I wish I had spent more days at the office.'" As another, "Stop and smell the roses." Some businesses now encourage employees to volunteer in the community, to have outside interests and to look after their health, including stress levels, but such employees are often middle or top management, leaving people on assembly lines and the like with as boring and stressful jobs as ever. Remember "Leisure Studies" as a promising field in, I think, the 1980s? For a brief while, we assumed that computers would take over much of our work, and we'd have a lot of free time. But surveys now show that many Americans routinely work more hours than ever, and our vacations are shorter than Europeans'. Our hearts, both physical and cultural, need more R & R & R: rest, recreation, and revitalization. The heart's pulsing cycle is a miniature model of systole and diastole, effort and relaxation. Happy people are often healthy people, and even happy people with health dilemmas do better than unhappy people with them. A recent Johns Hopkins study followed 586 healthy people who each had a sibling with heart problems at an early age; persons with positive outlooks were only one half as likely to have heart trouble as those with negative outlooks. "A cheerful heart is good medicine, but a downcast spirit dries up the bones."

The epidemiological approach suggests we should care for all of our hearts, a corporate sense of wellness, a commonwealth. In discussing the Giant Heart in Philadelphia, we considered the notion of *philakardia,* a love of hearts which would motivate us to care for our individual hearts and for the hearts of all creatures, especially humans. As a society, what can we do to support heart health, not only through adequate health care but also through preventive measures such as recreation, resources for aesthetic and spiritual experience, and healthy cities?

The second interpretation of "synthetic multiplicity" has two layers of meaning, the natural and the social. Our hearts have kinship with other mammals (whose four-chambered hearts are structurally similar) and other living creatures in nature. Their hearts are equally mortal, by individual and by species; indeed, their fates and ours are intertwined. Away from my urban setting and my sedentary job, I found the nature of the Rockies to be rich and primal, with roots millions of years old and patterns of loss and renewal that also echoed, in immense scale, the systole and diastole of all pumping hearts. As I considered the mountains, animals, and weather patterns, I felt more a part of nature—not just some visitor or tourist, and I could see nature as the matrix from which all creatures have come. By their basic atoms, our hearts are linked to the earth, to deer and bear, to shrimp and eagles, to forests and volcanoes. In other words, *we belong* to the home of the earth, the *oikos* that is a root for the word "ecology," whether the solid ground of Steve's cabin and tree farm or Kay's dirt of the rodeo arena. Belongingness is clearly a concept opposite to alienation, loneliness, hunger, or despair. A gratuitous but nonetheless suggestive anagram of the word *heart* is the word *earth,* and we've seen earlier that the words *human* and *humus* are directly related. For all the abstractions we place upon hearts, they are, in some ways, simple objects that do one job extremely well, but they also link efficiently to all the systems of our bodies and link symbolically to the heartedness of all creatures and to the nature of all nature.

As we saw in the passages above on animal hearts and Yellowstone, nature is wonderfully complex and interlinked. The hearts of animals and humans developed through evolution, a process of immense length and implausible complexity, including different versions of very early humans and bizarre events: diebacks of species, changes in world climate, volcanic events, even collisions with asteroids. From this chaotic but wondrous chronology, our hearts emerged as gifts, state-of-the-art organs custom-designed for active humans. The meat of the heart is largely muscle, muscle that will work a long time with little care, but that may work longer and assuredly better if it is exercised. Dr. Knapp and Doreen (and many others) have spoken of each of us as managers of our own health, humans who know the earth of their bodies, their own local humus. Contemporary lifestyles of sitting in cars, sitting in chairs, sitting at desks, riding in elevators, using "labor-saving devices," watching TV, and eating fatty foods make it difficult to keep our hearts healthy; as an academic, I know all too well the sedentary lifestyle and why the phrase "Ivory Tower" can accurately suggest a removal from the earth, from reality. American children are now said to have an epidemic of obesity as they play video games, lose their recesses at school (insurance reasons), and consume high-calorie drinks and snacks. In contrast, we recall the rodeo clowns—athletic, active, and savvy; they are men of the soil, clownish, and cloddish, who use humor as a way to confront danger. The rodeo clowns show us how to live in the dirt and how to save lives of the riders, in a strange parallel with medical doctors. There is another resonance of *humus,* however, the rotting vegetation that makes soil rich, deaths that make new lives possible. The Yellowstone volcano eruption blew away a mountain and created a wonderland. Stars had to explode to give us most of the elements in the universe. When we die, our materials will once again feed the earth—immediately, if we are cremated—or eventually, even if our bodies are embalmed and locked in concrete vaults.

The conclusion I draw is that the heart each of us has is a part of nature, a gift or even a miracle that has been created by nature, and will, after death, return to nature. It is natural to have hearts. Most readers (and the writer) of this book are urban; we have many advantages to our city life, but there are some losses also. To live optimally with our hearts, we would need to recreate benefits of a nonurban lifestyle, a parallel to Dr. Grant's medical tricks to help sick hearts act as they did when they were healthy.

Returning to the social meanings of the "synthetic multiplicity" of the heart, we can recall our discussion of Bellah's work, including the notion that there's no such thing as a private citizen. Without repeating arguments for a common good (or a commonwealth), we can say that supportive social interactions positively influence our mental and physical health, our hearts included. As we recognize and support the humanity of other people, they recognize and support our own, and our empathy goes up, and our stress goes down. Our four heart patients in this book all drew sustenance from social links and often sought ways to support others. The heart patients in the rehab lab and the Mended Hearts Club members gave support to each other. Whether our hearts are cheerful or not can influence our blood pressure, our behaviors with food and exercise, our self-image, and, in general, our motivation to take care of our physical being. In short, the cultural senses of the heart (and our individual versions of these) influence our physical hearts—which, in turn, can influence our emotions and general outlook on life.

Overlapping Circles of Medicine and Culture

When I started this project, I had the vague hope that I could create a magical and total synthesis of the two approaches to the heart, the scientific and the cultural; I could be a modern-day Pico della Mirandola, the "Great Reconciler," who hoped to put Greek philosophers and Christianity into a single, larger system. But a complete merger of the two is impossible and, I think, undesirable. Science needs to be technical and sophisticated in maximal ways; literature, the arts, and other humanistic fields need to explore limits of form and exercise freely all mental faculties. Science and humanism should extend their own specializations and boundaries but they can also be in dialogue, can overlap, can interpenetrate. In the 1950s, C. P. Snow called for a rapprochement of the two cultures of science and humanism, and, in many ways, this is happening, for example, in the new field of medical humanities (including bioethics, literature and medicine, history and medicine, anthropology and medicine), which has provided ways for the two areas to talk with each other.

It would be tempting to suggest that all persons in all places should have all perspectives—scientific, cultural, social, and personal—in mind, but this clearly isn't possible or even desirable. Within a healthy society, however, it would be desirable to have all such perspectives. We need our scientists, our theorists, our artists, our lab technicians, our foresters, our manufacturers, and so on. Ideally, they should be in conversation, learning from each other, so that each role can be informed and enriched by several others, so that they support the health of all humans and the health of the planet.

How can we best live with our hearts? As I look over the Alcove Model, it seems to me that there are many concepts to chose from as we perceive and interpret our hearts. I don't intend to contemplate these every day—that would constitute an unhealthy obsession. Rather, when I think of my heart, I'll have models that may interpret it positively, making it less likely that I'll automatically think of negative views (the pump about to break, the place where my neuroses dwell). I'm suggesting that there is a psychological parallel to Gresham's Law of money applicable to psychic space: very simply, good thoughts can push out bad thoughts. While the four areas of the Alcove Model are reminiscent of the four chambers of the heart, I'm not banking on this similarity as necessary or sufficient. My four patients illustrated many aspects of the heart, and I'm confident others may and will be considered, especially as science continues to evolve. Technology, such as artificial hearts, might be still another alcove to draw in. Genetics and the new field of pharmacogenetics could be another. One interesting new direction is the emerging science of energy medicine. According to James L. Oschman, the heart produces various kinds of energy (with the appropriate measuring device in parentheses): sound (audiogram), pressure (kymogram), heat pulse (thermogram), and an electromagnetic pulse (electrocardiogram, magnetocardiogram). The electromagnetic pulse of the heart is about fifty times that of the brain, making the heart the most powerful electromagnetic organ in the body. Taken all together, these forms of energy have been described as a dynamic energy system which may communicate through the vasculature to every cell in the body (*Energy Medicine: The Scientific Basis* [Edinburgh: Churchill Livingstone, 2000]). In a more applied approach, the Institute of HeartMath (Boulder Creek, Calif.) studies the heart's beating pulses, believing that a coherent pulse (with limited variability) shows a healthy, nonstressed person. In his later book, *Energy Medicine in Therapeutics and Human Performance* (Edinburgh: Butterworth Heinemann, 2003), Oschman mentions studies of cellular memory that may explain reports that patients receiving transplanted hearts also receive memories from the donor. According to the new field of neurocardiology, the heart is in continuous and sophisticated conversation with the brain, especially the emotional-cognitive portion. Thus love may, in some sense, be based in our beating hearts, just as valentine hearts always said it was.

Another version of intersecting circles comes to me from the night sky. In Montana, the clean mountain air and a minimum of light scatter led me to do some stargazing; except for the chill, winter is a great season for stars. The constellations are among the brightest and most dramatic: Taurus, the Pleiades, Orion, Canis Major, all parading across the sky. Stargazing guides tell of wonderful things. For instance, our sun is an average star in size and temperature, between the mammoth red giants near the end of their lives (for example Betelgeuse, the reddish star on Orion's shoulder) and young blue-white stars of immense heat (for example, Rigel, diagonally across from Betelgeuse, at Orion's foot). Rigel is a double star, two stars circling each other, but you see this phenomenon only through a telescope. My naive view is that single stars are points of light, but the guides say over half of them are double, some even triple. From this dynamic image I find a celestial metaphor, the cultural heart and the biological heart as two stars, circling each other. Depending on our viewpoint, we see one, the other, both together as one, or neither—as in the invisible stars of the daytime. Our viewpoint of the heart can change with our interest, attention, state of health, or with technology—even as simple a tool as a stethoscope. The two stars can compete for our attention or they can illuminate and enrich each other. If we focus on the heart values of our cultural heart, we can celebrate how the biological heart maintains our lives, our awareness, our thought. Further, we can affirm some of the heart values we found in our language (center, wisdom, courage, love, eros). We can lower our stress by feeling at home in nature and with our fellow creatures, human and nonhuman.

If we focus on the health of our biological heart, our mental attitudes and our behaviors can support or detract from how we partner with the wonderful organs in our chests. If we see the two working in synergy, we can manage how we live with them—selectively and individually. "Selectively" means, for me, attention to our hearts as needed, neither an obsession nor a complete denial. "Individually" means—as the heart patients in this book have shown—that we each make our own package, drawing on the many resources now available, fabulous riches compared to the knowledge of earlier times. As we lower our stress and find meaning in our lives, our physical hearts are more likely to stay healthy.

One resource now available is *The Okinawa Program* (New York: Clarkson Potter, 2001), a sizeable but accessible volume by Bradley J. Wilcox, M.D., M.Sc., a geriatrics fellow at Harvard; D. Craig Wilcox, Ph.D., a medical anthropologist at Okinawa Prefectural University; and Makoto Suzuki, M.D., Ph.D., a cardiologist and geriatrician at Okinawa International University. All three are investigators in a twenty-five-year Okinawa Centenarian Study, a Japanese Ministry of Health-sponsored study of the world's healthiest and longest-lived people. (Speaking of twin stars: the Wilcoxes are identical twins.) The subtitle provides a good summary: "How the World's Longest-Lived People Achieve Everlasting Health—and How You Can Too." The basic news is not surprising; our health—especially our cardiac health—is optimized by four factors: (1) a healthy diet emphasizing fruits, vegetables, and grains, de-emphasizing meats, dairy, fats, and salt; (2) a healthy lifestyle resulting in lean, active bodies; (3) excellent psychospiritual health that leads to low stress, and (4) integrative health care (western and eastern). While we see such lessons regularly (including in this book), what I find powerful in *The Okinawa Program* is the weight of scientific evidence for each of the claims, the clarity of the author's presentation, and the interviews and anecdotes about individual, active, and elderly Okinawans who make the lessons dramatic, giving us persuasive images—mythic guides, we might even say—of healthy old age. All four factors will help motivate me to follow the advice of the book, to enjoy the binary hearts of my body.

Mortality/Vitality

Intellectual fashions of the Renaissance, the Enlightenment, nineteenth-century positivism, and twentieth-century pragmatism tend to ignore the emotions. School curricula (largely aimed at skill development) and college and university courses (now often aimed at job training) do little with the emotions, except for some courses in the arts. And yet emotion has a lot to do with our physical health, cardiac health in particular, as we have seen. The human nature of the mind can influence the human nature of the body, and vice versa. What did my Uncle Hector feel, alone in his car following his heart attack, with pain crushing his chest and sweat dripping down his face? As fellow humans, we can make some good guesses. He was scared . . . terrified. He feared death and—perhaps even more—debility, crippling weakness in a society that celebrates (and expects) perfect health.

The red heart on a fencer's costume suggests the mortality we all share; the human heart is, among other things, a symbol of death. We've known for millennia that when the pulse is gone, the person is dead. Our hearts will stop someday, for reasons we can only partially control, an ill-defined *terminus ad quem* toward which we are headed. I remember a workshop exercise in which each participant was directed to write his or her obituary, picking the age of death and describing the life story up to that point. (I found the assignment disturbing—as if the words might, in fact, predict my demise; fortunately there was a less threatening alternative: we could merely list our general personal aims.) Still, if I am to die in ten years, how should I spend them? In five years? In one year? What personal philosophy or religion might I explore to illuminate this world and, possibly, the next? Illness, accidents, and close calls reawaken our attention to such questions, but then we typically subside into the habits and pressures (or perceived pressures) of daily life.

Paradoxically, the human heart is also a symbol of life. Each beat we feel in our chests, wrists, or necks tells us that the magnificent heart and many other wonderful systems are working in our bodies, making our thoughts, emotions, and behaviors possible. Vitality and mortality are mirror images, two sides of a Janus figure, our malleable and ever-changing lives and the undefined yet certain deaths we will someday encounter. How will we live within—and even celebrate—this vitality? How can we enjoy the earth and its creatures, our fellow beings, resources—whether slender or generous—that we have to work with? As humans, we are limited in time and space, but we reach, in various ways, for the stars. Each of us makes his or her own assemblage, consciously or unconsciously. One formulation comes from an ancient Hebrew:

> Go, eat your bread with enjoyment, and drink your wine with a merry heart; for God has long ago approved what you do. Let your garments always be white; do not let oil be lacking on your head. Enjoy life with the wife whom you love, all the days of your vain life that are given you under the sun, because that is your portion in life and in your toil at which you toil under the sun. Whatever your hand finds to do, do with your might. . . . (Ecclesiastes 9:7–10)

A modern version would speak of a husband or significant other(s), and the imagery of food and clothes might change, but the *merry heart* seems as important now, as pivotal now, as it did centuries ago.

Journeys

I have enjoyed my journey from Florida to Montana and back, my journey speaking with patients, doctors, researchers, my journey in various texts, literary and scientific. The dictionary tells me that the root of the word "journey" is the French *jour* or "day," meaning how far a person might travel in a day—a wonderfully elastic concept nowadays as we consider that humans might be bushwhacking through dense forest or speeding over continents and oceans on jet airplanes. The notion of travel within a time frame is, however, a basic and universal description of our lives from birth to death. As I review our four heart patients, I see a progression that I did not notice until near the end of my study. Michael, the young man in his twenties, represents the robust strengths of athletic youth and the search for work appropriate to his talents and training. Kay, about a decade older, is more the strategic survivor, an endurance athlete according to her own definition. Steve, at fifty-one, is a midlife person who has redesigned his living habits and his mental habits. At ninety-one, Johnnie is the ultimate survivor, a man living with support and with deficits, but in a mental framework that makes sense of his life past and present and his life in a world yet to come. Each of these has come to terms with his or her heart—medically and culturally—through his or her own synthesis. Different in age and overall health, they cannot share one single formula. One feature they all share, however, is their mortality, which each of them looked at squarely; because of this confrontation, all made decisions that helped give their lives meaning.

My journey is temporarily over; my course of study is at an end; it's time for a tentative conclusion. Biomedical understanding of the heart will continue ever forward, as Dr. Duran and others make new discoveries, find new surgical techniques, create better drugs; the heart is a magnet for the thoughts and skills of humans. Heart research will continue at many clinics and labs around the world. If a scientist were to solve coronary artery disease tomorrow, surely a Nobel Prize would be appropriate, not to mention the thanks of millions of patients and their physicians. Will cultural attention to the heart and heart values continue? I can't be as sure, although I certainly hope so. Can we give more attention to heart values, including compassion for the poor (see Barbara Ehrenreich's *Nickel and Dimed: On (Not) Getting by in America* [New York: Metropolitan Books, 2001]), care for the health of our citizens (for example, adequate health-care insurance) and all the citizens of the world (for instance, adequate funding for nutrition and HIV/AIDS), care for the health of our forests and fields, our cities and governments, our streams, rivers, and oceans—all these can profit from attention to essence, wisdom, courage, love, and emotion.

Our informants—Michael, Kay, Steve—will continue their lives in various ways. As for Michael and his father, they did climb Mt. Kilimanjaro; Michael sent me a postcard showing the snow-covered volcano they climbed. Kay continues her job and her healthy routine. Steve's church and his life both prosper. Johnnie was the first to find out about heaven; he departed this earth on September 9, 2001. The rest of us will eventually die, myself included. But I now have a better repertory of ways to live with my heart until then, to enjoy it and to take care of it, as well as a better sense of how to live with the hearts of others, to enjoy them, to take care of them, to love them. All that is certain is that my heart will someday stop working. I can admit that and, for the moment anyway, accept it; my trip to the hospital with chest pain was, perhaps, a dress rehearsal. (The episode of chest pain I experienced was finally assessed as a possible coronary artery spasm or, more likely, an esophagitis caused by drinking orange juice on an empty stomach.)

The heart seems more wonderful than when I began, an organ that belongs to all humanity, and to most of our fellow creatures on this earth. Whatever fears and anxieties I was housing in my heart are either gone or temporarily residing elsewhere. All pains and twinges in my chest have gone away. I am no longer afraid of my grandmother's heart trouble, or my uncle's heart attack, ghosts I have dispelled.

What, then, is the human heart? It is many things, depending on the point of view of the observer, the definer, the language user. As the heart itself is "avid" for certain radiopharmaceuticals, so the human mind is avid for meanings. From the Mary of Luke's gospel to Faust, from the Renaissance explorers to today's biochemists looking at heart tissue, we want to know about our world, our bodies, and the meanings that give life context and value.

One December evening in Missoula, near the end of our stay in Montana, my wife and I were preparing to return to Florida. We'd seen only light snow so far, but it was often chilly and windy—and thoroughly, stygianly dark by 5:00 P.M. Dixie McLaughlin, from the institute, and her husband Gary invited us to dinner at their house on the edge of town. After eating, we put on our swimsuits and raced across a freezing, dark patio to their hot tub, where we luxuriated in bone-warming water. We looked out across the lights of Missoula in one direction and, on the other side, up Pattee Canyon, home to deer, cats, and bear—all with their hearts, some awake and prowling, some asleep, some in adaptive hypothermia. We couldn't really see the canyon in the dark, but we could see the top edge of it, where the ponderosa pines were silhouetted against the starry night sky. And what a sky! The stars were strewn lavishly from horizon to horizon, uncountable stars from the brightest to the barely visible, so many that the major constellations were overwhelmed and hard to discern. But there was the Milky Way, a myriad of stars in an undulating stripe roughly from north to south, our own galaxy seen edge on, our heavenly address. And, yes, Orion with his dogs, and Taurus, and the Pleiades. I remembered a remark by my mother, "You know, people just don't see the stars anymore." She knew fabulous stars from childhood summers in rural Michigan several decades ago; now a city dweller, she sees only the handful allowed by air pollution and light scatter. Perhaps we all need star therapy, a chance to be dazzled by their number and the huge spaces and times they imply, the opportunity to see ourselves as part of something larger, the grace to consider that we are encompassed by (and were created within) a universe of colossal size and, still, cosmic order. Indeed, the word "consider" has the Latin root of "sidus," meaning "star," suggesting that close observation and studied interpretation in large contexts are necessary, that humans need space and time—thinking all night?—to make their considerations. The Big Bang Theory considers that the stars gave us all the elements for this earth, for these many bodies, for these many hearts. I think of the stars surrounding us night and day, always and forever, the magma under Yellowstone (and under us wherever we stand), and the magnificent hearts beating within us, as natural as any part of nature, all made of the same atoms and molecules, all evidence of meaning and order for us to consider, to cherish, to revere.

Index